YOGA

anytime *anyplace* *anybody*

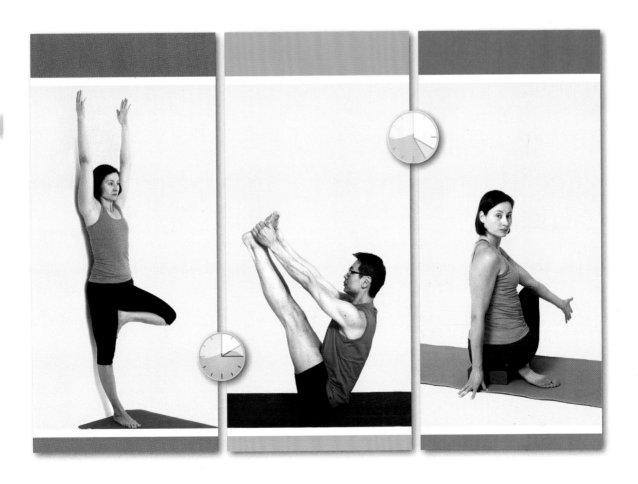

Published in 2013 by

media*Eight*

Media Eight Publishing India Private Limited

302-A, ABW Tower, MG Road
Gurgaon 122002, India

Tel: +91 (0)124 4040017

ISBN: 978-81-7314-265-9

Printed in India

YOGA

anytime

anyplace

anybody

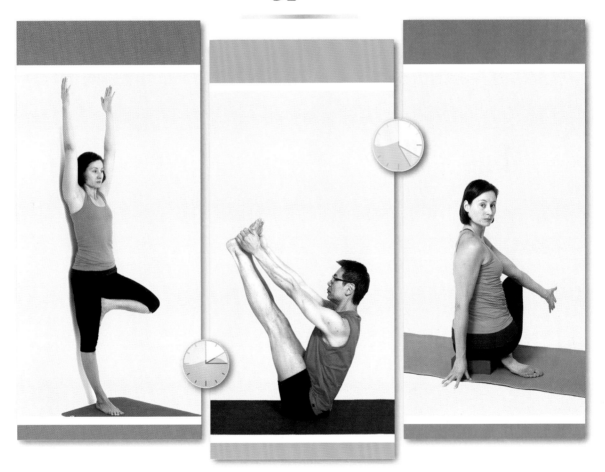

RACHEL GRAVES

media *S*ight

CONTENTS

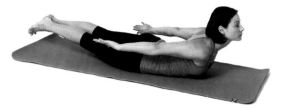

69 | Medium Programmes

CONTENTS

CONTENTS

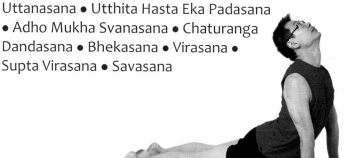

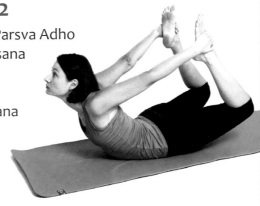
CONTENTS

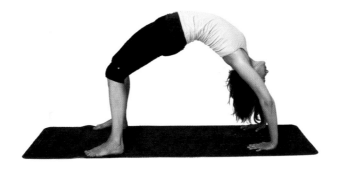

Yoga makes you feel good

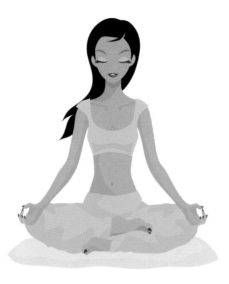

There are many, well documented advantages of yoga, but the most compelling reason for practising it is also the most simple: it makes you feel great.

Practising yoga can improve strength, stamina and flexibility. It can encourage better sleep and improve digestion. It can help with weight management, improve muscle tone and increase coordination and physical self reliance. Yoga can improve posture, reduce stress levels and encourage concentration.

Fifteen minutes of yoga daily, or whenever you can manage it, can provide benefits which are disproportionate to the time expended.

Both physically and mentally yoga can provide immense benefits – all of which are achievable in very short periods of time.

Despite our best intentions, many of us never quite manage to maintain a regular programme of exercise, citing either a lack of time or space to do so. However, you do not need an abundance of either for yoga to be a part of your life. Ten minutes of yoga a day really does count. Also, yoga can be done anywhere. You can practise in your bathroom, in your lounge, or in your bedroom. You can even practise with other people around, if that is the only way you can manage it. So instead of feeling that you can't fit your life around yoga, fit yoga into your life.

Yoga requires nothing of you except whatever time you choose to give it. Whatever stage you are at in your life, and no matter what you are faced with, yoga is constant, and undemanding.

If you are seeking better sleep or digestion, or relaxation and a sense of well being, yoga can help. If you are looking to fit some physical activity into a life that already seems too full of commitments, or if it is merely stretching you require after some other form of exercise, yoga can provide a solution. If you are looking to strengthen your body, or develop stamina, or improve your concentration, or become more self aware, or start a meditation practice, yoga can help you achieve these things.

Yoga mobilises the joints of the body, improving flexibility. Strength and stamina are developed, and the muscles are toned and lengthened. Coordination is improved, enabling the practitioner to become more self reliant physically – something that becomes more pertinent as we age. Posture is corrected, so the internal organs are able to function efficiently.

> *Whatever you are looking for in terms of exercise or health, yoga can contribute in a positive way.*

INSTRUCTIONS FOR CORRECT PRACTICE

SAFETY

A yoga mat is best to practise on, as it will ensure you don't slip. If you don't use one, be aware of how you place your hands and feet, and only use non-slippery surfaces to practise on. If using furniture in your practice, make sure it is fixed or lodged in such a way that it will not move.

ALIGNMENT

Correct alignment in yoga is vital, so that you receive the maximum benefit from each posture, and don't do damage to yourself. Although this book is a guide to the basics of improving your alignment, if you can attend a class as well, then do so – a well trained and observant teacher will correct you in a way that you cannot achieve for yourself.

HOW TO USE THIS BOOK

This book is designed to be used by anybody. You do not need to have practised yoga before, but if you have, this book can help you develop or progress your own practice.

1

The book is arranged into timed sequences of postures, starting with the shortest. The sequences are designed to be done around the home: on page 27, you can find suggestions of where they can be practised, using various common household items as props. When you become familiar with how to practise, and what props you need, you should be able to adapt your practice to other places.

TIMING

The short sequences are made up of just three or four postures, designed to be done in ten or fifteen minutes. The medium length sequences have five to seven postures, designed to be done in twenty or twenty-five minutes. The longer sequences have between eight to twelve postures, and are designed to be done in thirty-five to forty-five minutes. However, the timing for the postures is a rough guide, not something you have to stick to rigidly. For example, some postures are single-sided, which will take less time to practise than the double-sided postures. Some postures have optional variations, which you can skip if you're pushed for time. Also, if you're a beginner, it may take you time to work out how to get into the postures, and then when you are in them, a few minutes might feel like a very long time indeed. Don't worry too much about the timing. The aim is to be in the posture for between two and five minutes, but to start with, just do what feels manageable. As you get more used to practising, you'll find you can hold postures for longer.

Sometimes it can feel very daunting to contemplate doing yoga on your own for forty minutes. Ten minutes, though, isn't so overwhelming. You might find that you're more comfortable doing three short sequences, either together or spaced out during the day, rather than one long one.

BUILDING UP YOUR UNDERSTANDING

More detail about the postures is given as the programmes increase in length – so the short programmes start with the basics only, and the longer ones provide more information on the subtler actions. By starting with the short programmes and working up, you'll increase your understanding of the postures. Remember that it takes time for the brain and the body to absorb new instructions. Sometimes you can hear or read the same instruction hundreds of times, and it makes no sense. Don't worry too much about this. To begin with, concentrate on getting the basics right – that way your practice will be a safe one. The subtler instructions will become clear in their own time, when the body is ready. When you have been practising on the basics for a while, approach those new instructions simply by taking your attention to the area of the body in question. Gradually, and with practice, your body will understand the basic actions in yoga well enough to connect to the new ones.

BREATHING

Breathe normally, through the nose, throughout your practice. Try not to hold the breath, even in the more challenging postures. If you have a blocked nose, do your best to breathe through the nose, but if that is impossible, breathe through the mouth.

THE SEQUENCE OF POSTURES WITHIN EACH PROGRAMME

Do the postures in the sequence laid out in each programme. They are designed to work the body in a particular way, and if you change the order that the postures appear in, it can be jarring for the body. Notwithstanding this, the sequences can be practised one after the other, if you choose to do so. They are complete within themselves, so postures still shouldn't be missed out, but you can practise any of the sequences together, in any order. Also, you can repeat postures if you choose to, keeping within the sequence laid out. So if you feel that a particular posture is helpful, or that you're starting to understand it better, then feel free to do it again. This can be very beneficial, as it allows the body to remember actions and build on them.

Regardless of the focus of a yoga practice, there is a certain sequence which, when followed, ensures that the body is worked and mobilised in such a way that is beneficial. So, the spine is always lengthened before any twists or forward or backward bends are practised. Backward bends are both demanding and invigorating, so should be integrated into the middle of a practice, to allow the spine first to be warmed up and then the mind and body to be brought to a quieter state afterwards: this is particularly important for evening practice, before going to bed. Forward bends are restful for the mind, so are often done towards the end of a practice. If working on both forward and backward bends in one session, the spine needs to be brought into a neutral position in between, as it can be uncomfortable to go straight from a strong backward bend into a forward bend. Twists are very good for bringing the spine back to a neutral position. Gentler postures that open the body are practised before stronger ones. So before working into Padmasana or lotus, postures that open the hips and pelvis are always practised first, so that the joints are warmed and mobilised. Working into strong postures too quickly can result in the body being strained or damaged.

DIFFICULTY OF THE POSTURES

In the shorter sequences, postures are introduced with support and modifications so that they are fairly gentle. In the longer sequences, full postures are shown, plus more challenging ones. If, when moving on to the longer sequences, you find that the full postures are too challenging, you can always go back to the easier version of the postures that you have practised from the shorter programmes. However, if you find that you are struggling with all the postures in the longer sequences, just go back to the shorter sequences, which are easier. When you feel that the shorter sequences are coming better, you can try the longer sequences again, with their more challenging postures. Never force yourself into postures. If you force the body to go further than it is ready to go, you can cause injury. Find an appropriate balance for you – it's fine to challenge your body in order to progress, but it is important to do so without strain.

WHEN TO MODIFY YOUR PRACTICE

- If you are unwell and don't feel like practising yoga, then don't. Often the body knows what it needs. Learn to listen to it.
- If you are feeling over-tired, emotionally fragile or run down, for whatever reason, sometimes a recuperative practice can be beneficial. This means seated and supine postures, done with support to allow the body to find the correct position without straining.
- If you are tired, a restful sequence can open and mobilise the body without strain.
- When you have been unwell, but have recovered enough to feel ready to begin your practice again, a recuperative sequence should be followed. This will help improve your energy levels and mobilise the body, but will be gentler than a regular practice, so as to avoid straining or over-taxing the body.
- For women, if you are at the beginning of your period, practise the recuperative sequence. After this, practise the restful sequences. Towards the middle or end of your period, or when you feel your energy levels start to improve, practise the restorative sequences. If the restorative sequences are too much, go back to the recuperative or restful sequences.

RECUPERATIVE SEQUENCES

S3 {with the arm variations in Virasana omitted} ; *L3*

RESTFUL SEQUENCES

S3; L2

RESTORATIVE SEQUENCES

S1; S2; S4; M1 {with Trikonasana and Ardha Chandrasana practised against a wall}

CONTRAINDICATIONS –
WHEN YOU SHOULD *NOT* PRACTISE CERTAIN POSTURES

There shouldn't be any sharp pain in yoga – if there is, then something is going wrong, and you should stop. Equally, the body doesn't like doing things that are uncomfortable, so know the difference between something being painful and something causing discomfort. Often the posture you want to release most quickly because it's uncomfortable is often the one that is most beneficial for you to persevere with. So just be sensitive in your practice, so that you can progress without injuring yourself.

Some medical conditions and injuries mean that certain postures will need to be adapted, or not practised at all. If you have a medical condition, you should consult your doctor before starting yoga, and then if given approval to practise, you should work under the guidance of a well-qualified teacher, to ensure that you work in a way that is not detrimental to your health.

ASTHMA: Yoga opens the chest and improves the posture of the upper body, which can benefit the health of the lungs. However, some postures which constrict the front body can be unhelpful for those who suffer from asthma. Avoid the following postures in this book or practise them with a teacher: Paripurna Navasana, Marichyasana 1 (as a forward bend) and Malasana.

BACK AND NECK INJURIES: This depends on the nature of the injury, but if you have a back or neck injury, it is better to work with supervision to ensure no further damage is done. If you have back ache, which is not due to a medical problem or injury, practise the recuperative and restful short sequences to begin with, concentrating on improving your alignment and lengthening your spine. Forward bends might be too strong for the back; in which case upright seated variations of those postures can be practised instead.

WRIST INJURIES: Depending on the severity of the problem, you should avoid all postures where weight is held in the hands – such as Adho Mukha Svanasana (downward dog). Postures where the wrist is bent strongly, such as Paschima Namaskarasana, should also be avoided. If the injury is mild and exercise of the wrist has been recommended, just work gently to begin with: practise Adho Mukha Svanasana with the hands on a chair *(Image 2)*, for example, which moves the weight back into the feet, and out of the wrists. Practise Urdhva Baddhanguliyasana (interlacing the fingers and taking the hands above the head) in Tadasana or Virasana to mobilise the wrists, but without forcing the action or causing yourself pain.

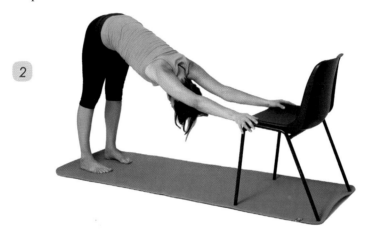

ANKLE INJURIES: If the problem is severe, avoid sitting on the ankles, such as in Virasana and Adho Mukha Virasana. If stretching the ankle gently has been advised to improve healing, only do these postures with padding under the ankle *(Image 3)*. Depending on the nature of the injury, you may also need to avoid postures which require strength and flexibility in the ankles, such as Adho Mukha Svanasana, Utthita Parsvakonasana, Parsvottanasana,

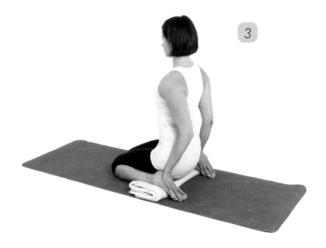

Prasarita Padottanasana and Malasana. Other postures may be practised with support for the ankles – such as Supta Baddha Konasana, Baddha Konasana, Swastikasana and Supta Swastikasana.

HEART PROBLEMS: Consult your doctor first. If the condition is not a benign one, you should practise with a teacher rather than on your own. Back bends can be stimulating to the heart, and forward bends restful, but you may need individual guidance depending on the nature of the problem.

HIGH BLOOD PRESSURE: Work with a teacher who can guide you. In particular, you should avoid Marichyasana (twists), Parsvottanasana, Utthita Trikonasana and Ustrasana.

LOW BLOOD PRESSURE: Same as for high blood pressure, plus Tadasana, Vrksasana, Ardha Chandrasana and Utkatasana.

KNEE INJURIES OR PROBLEMS: If the problem is not severe, always do kneeling postures on a soft surface: have your mat on a carpet or rug, or have a blanket or towel on your mat. In bent leg postures, always take a belt or rope into the back of the knee, pulling it well forward on both sides of the joint and holding it firmly in front of the knee cap before bending the knee.

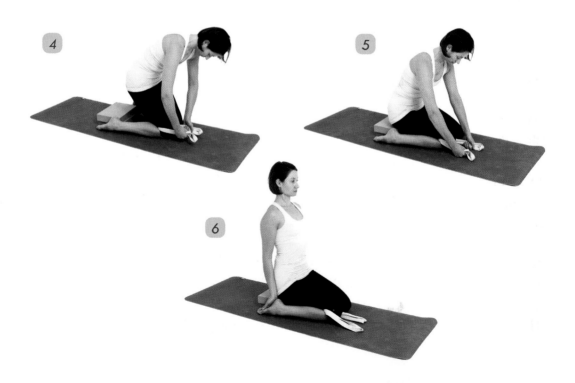

In kneeling postures such as Virasana, take a belt behind the knee joint and sit up on a support to ensure the knee is not strained *(Images 4, 5 and 6)*.

Ustrasana (camel) can be practised if the problem is not severe and kneeling up gives no pain – but make sure you kneel on something soft. In Swastikasana, Supta Swastikasana, Baddha Konasana and Supta Baddha Konasana, take support under the knees and thighs so that the knees are not strained *(Image 8)*. Avoid Padmasana.

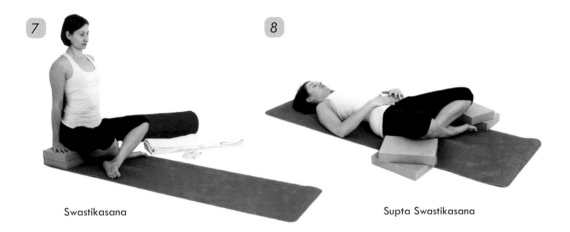

Swastikasana　　　　　　　　　　　　Supta Swastikasana

In standing postures, make sure the front thigh muscles and kneecaps are well lifted. This will give support to the knee joint. If you find that standing balancing postures put too much strain on the knee, then avoid these.

If the problem is severe, consult a doctor before you practise, and make sure you attend classes with a teacher as well as practising on your own, to ensure that the knees are being placed and supported correctly in the various postures.

MENSTRUATION: Avoid strong abdominal work such as Ardha and Paripurna Navasana and Urdhva Prasarita Padasana. Avoid all twists, such as Marichyasana, all standing twists such as Parivrtta Ardha Chandrasana, and all supine twists such as Jathara Parivartanasana and Supta Padanghustasana 3. Avoid postures where the hips are raised above the line of the head, such as Adho Mukha Svanasana, or where the legs are raised, such as Viparita Karani.

PREGNANCY: Postures that require strong abdominal work and most twists should not be practised at all during pregnancy, and most other postures are modified in some way, to support the body as it changes. **Because these modifications couldn't be shown in this book, this book should not be used as a guide for practice during**

pregnancy. If you are new to yoga, you should practise with a teacher who is qualified in prenatal teaching. If you are an experienced practitioner, make sure that you speak to a teacher to find out how you should modify your own practice to ensure it is both safe and beneficial during your pregnancy.

WHEN TO PRACTISE – EATING AND DRINKING

Generally, it is advisable not to eat or drink one to two hours before you practise. However, if you're trying to fit yoga into your life at odd moments, then this can be a challenge. If you have just eaten, the following postures can be done at any time:

SEATED	STANDING	SUPINE
Virasana	Tadasana	Supta Virasana
Swastikasana		Supta Baddha Konasana
Baddha Konasana		(Support under the back
Dandasana		and head may be needed
Upavistha Konasana		to ensure that the action
(All upright, and all with		is not too strong on the
or without arm variations)		abdomen)

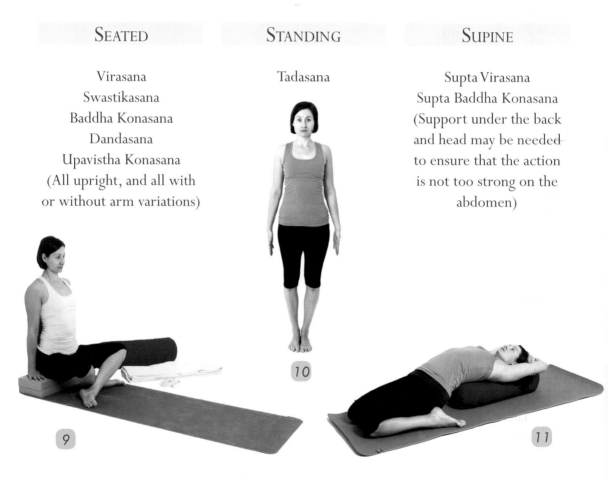

9   10   11

If you have eaten a snack or light meal, you might find that most of the postures are fine to practise, but you should avoid forward and backward bends, strong abdominal work, prone postures and twists.

Sequences which don't contain any of these actions are:
S1 S2 S3 S4 S5 S6 L3

PROBLEM SOLVING –
SEQUENCES TO HELP WITH PARTICULAR COMPLAINTS

Yoga can help with various general problems, such as troubled sleep, anxiety, lack of energy, abdominal discomfort and bloating, stiffness and aching muscles. The following list is a guide to finding the right sequence if you are suffering from any of these.

Disturbed sleep, anxiety, trouble getting to sleep, over-busy mind that requires calming	*M1 M3 L2*
Bloating, digestive discomfort including constipation, a need to stretch out the stomach	*S3 L3*
Stiff shoulders, tension headaches, hunched shoulders	*S1 M4 L1 L4*
Tired legs, poor circulation in the legs	*S3 S6*
General fatigue, aching muscles and physical tiredness (with a need to allow the body to recuperate)	*S3 L2 L3*
Lethargy or ennui (with a need to revitalise the body)	*M3 M4 M5 L1*
Stiffness in the joints – all sequences will help, but particularly	*S3 S5 M1 M2 M4 M5 M6 M7 L1 L2 L3*

USING PROPS

There are various reasons for using props: to improve alignment, to learn the correct action in a posture, for safety, and for comfort.

The following postures are all practised with props in some of the sequences in this book. Some progress towards the final posture, without using the prop, but you can always go back to using props if your body is not ready to move on, or if you feel you haven't understood the correct action fully. Feel free to work at your own pace.

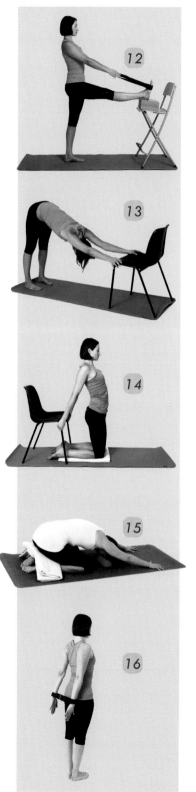

Having a belt around the foot in Supta Padangusthasana 1 and 2, and Utthita Hasta Padangusthasana
The belt is used
- when the foot can't be reached with the hand
- to get the correct alignment of the hips, tailbone and spine
- to ensure the legs are straight and the chest open

Placing the hands on a raised support for Adho Mukha Svanasana
- Improves the mobility in the shoulders, so the correct actions of the arms and shoulders can be learnt
- Moves the weight back into the heels

Holding a chair to work into Ustrasana
- Helps with the opening of the chest and the lift of the dorsal spine
- Allows the hands to learn to come into the final posture without losing the above actions

Supporting either the head or the buttocks in Adho Mukha Virasana
- Allows the head and neck to rest down, bringing quietness to the mind
- Enables the buttocks to extend down and connect with something (if not the heels), allowing the spine to lengthen from both ends

Tadasana with arm variations – using a belt
- Brings the arms closer together, in order to mobilise the shoulder joints and teach the correct action of the arms and shoulders

Using a wall for standing and seated postures
- Allows the alignment of the back body to be learnt
- In standing postures, enables the pupil to practise the posture without worrying about balance – therefore learning the correct actions first
- It is a more restful way of practising

Sitting up on a support for seated postures
- If there is stiffness in the legs or back and the back slumps, sitting up on a support encourages the sacrum to move in, and the spine to lift up
- It also allows the legs to release down

Supporting under the back body in Supta Virasana
- If the back doesn't come to the floor without causing pain in the knees or lumbar, taking support under the back body allows the back to rest down, rather than be in a halfway pose which has to be held with the arms. The essence of the posture can be felt and therefore improved

Support for the shins in kneeling postures: Supta Virasana, Virasana and Ustrasana:
- If the ankles are stiff and there is a large gap below the shin bones, it is difficult to connect this area with the floor, which is important for the extension of the spine. Placing support under the shins can encourage the frontal hip bones to lengthen more to the armpits, and the front body to extend to the head

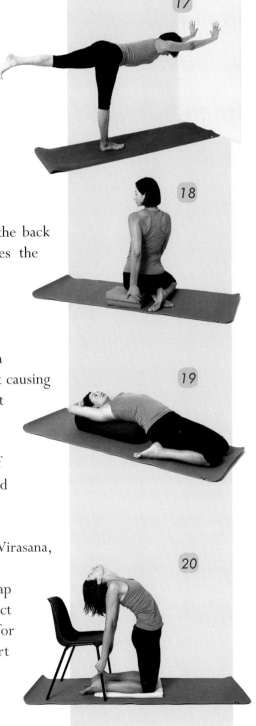

Support for the ankles in kneeling postures:
* If the ankles are stiff and kneeling is painful, placing some support under the ankles can relieve discomfort

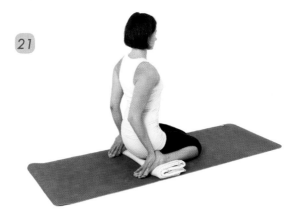

Support in the back of the knee in bent-legged postures (seated and some standing):
* Opens the back of the knee joint, relieving discomfort

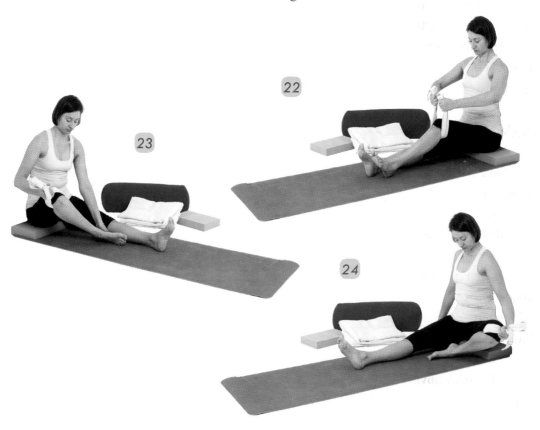

WHAT TO WEAR

Wear clothes that you can move in, and which are comfortable. Clothing should not restrict your actions – this includes clothes that are too tight, too baggy, too short, or have no stretch. It is distracting and irritating to have to untangle long trousers from around your feet, or adjust a T-shirt that has come untucked when you are practising.

When you're in a class, most teachers will request that you don't wear baggy clothing as it prevents them from seeing that the correct actions are being performed. Sometimes this also applies when you're practising on your own – to begin with, it can be useful to see that you have placed yourself correctly, before you can feel that you have.

Bare feet are best for yoga. Socks can slip, and with bare feet you can feel the feet fully.

A NOTE ABOUT THE PICTURES IN THIS BOOK

Many of the pictures in this book show the postures going to the right side – which traditionally is practised before the left side in yoga. Some pictures show going to the left side, either for clarity in the photo, or because a balance was required when the photographs were being taken. The written instructions always go to the right side first, regardless of the direction of the photo.

SAVASANA

Savasana, or corpse pose, is the primary relaxation posture in yoga, and is done at the end of almost every yoga practice. Often it is also used in between postures, to revive the body. It can also be done as a recuperative practice on its own, to allow the body to rest fully in the case of illness or fatigue – or simply after a hard day.

As it represents a hiatus between the physical practice and the rejoining of the outside world, Savasana can act as a kind of bridge between the body and the mind. Although it seems like just lying down – not a 'real' posture – it is precisely this absence of movement that is the most important quality of Savasana.

The most obvious benefit of Savasana is to allow the body to rest and recuperate after the physical work of the asana practice. Moreover, this resting time facilitates the assimilation of what has been learnt, so that a physical memory of the postures can be built up, separate to the intellectual memory of them.

What is more challenging than physical relaxation is for the mind to become quiet. In practising Savasana, one comes to accept that for the next few minutes, nothing will happen. The practitioner will not move, speak or shuffle (hopefully). At first, this is difficult – particularly so if we are practising on our own, without the discipline of someone else setting the schedule. Life is busy, and many of us have lost the art of doing nothing. Generally, we are thinking about what we should be doing, rather than appreciating what we are doing. However, this space, simply to be, is vital for the development of our yoga practice. Savasana eases us into a feeling of inner quietness and equanimity, without effort. So submit to it, just for a few minutes, and feel that in resting the body, we can train the mind also to find, accept and appreciate stillness.

Placing the body precisely for Savasana is important to get the maximum benefit from it. There are various ways of practising Savasana. The classic position is lying down flat, with the feet about hip bone width apart, and the arms just far enough away from the trunk that the side ribs do not touch the upper arms on the inhalation. This, and two other methods, are listed below.

If you find that your head tips back when you lie down, due to stiffness in the shoulders or upper spine, take some support under the back of the head.

Variation 1 – Classical Savasana

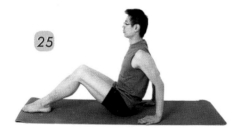

Start by sitting with the hands behind the hips and the knees bent *(Image 25)*. Lie down slowly, using the hands to lengthen the spine as you do so. Keep the knees bent. Move the muscles of the shoulders away from the ears, and lengthen the chest bone to the chin.

Allow the corners of the shoulders to fall to the floor, and the collar bones to separate. Lengthen the base of the back of the skull away from the shoulders, so that the skin of the face falls onto the

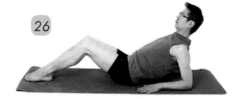

bones of the face, and the face becomes very quiet. Extend the flesh of the buttocks and the tailbone to the heels – you may need to lift your pelvis to do this *(Image 26)*. The lumbar should be long, and quiet. Release the abdomen down to the spine.

Extend the legs away one at a time, not taking them too wide, and allow the little toes to fall naturally to the sides, so the legs relax fully *(Image 29)*. Take the arms onto the floor beside you, with the palms facing up, to encourage the opening of the chest and ensure there is no sensory distraction to the fingertips.

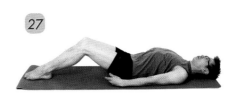

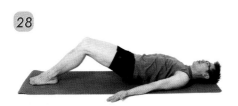

Generally the arms will be closer to the hips than the line of the shoulders: take them only as wide as you need to feel that the side ribs aren't disturbed as you inhale. If you take the arms too wide, some of the opening of the chest will be lost. Feel that you've placed yourself with mindfulness and attention to your alignment, so that you can relax the body completely.

The eyes can be open or closed, but if the eyes are open, the gaze should be soft. Let the eyes release down into their sockets. Let the tongue fall behind the lower teeth. Draw the inner ears in. Soften the senses, so the attention is drawn inward.

To come up, bend your knees by sliding the feet towards you, one at a time. Bend the arms so the hands come to rest on your body. Open the eyes slowly. Roll carefully on to your right side, keeping the knees bent. Let the top arm fall in front of the chest, so that the shoulders and hips are stacked on top of each other. Support the head with the lower arm, or a block or blanket. Press yourself up to sitting from your side, so that you don't disturb your back as you come up.

Note: You should come up out of all supine positions in this way.

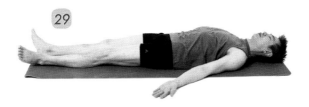

Variation 2 – with support under the legs

This is very restful for the back and the abdomen, and can be beneficial for those who find it uncomfortable to lie flat.

Take a wide support – such as a bolster, or a couple of rolled or folded blankets or towels – and place it under the back of the knees. From here, follow the instructions from the classical position, but when you extend the legs, feel that the back of the knees are resting on the support *(Image 30)*. The feet can be touching the floor, or slightly elevated, whichever you find most comfortable.

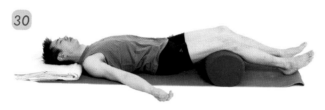

Variation 3 – with support under the spine

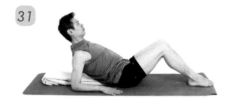

Have a pleated towel or blanket, long enough to rest your spine and head on. It needs to be about 15 cm wide so that you don't feel that you're going to fall off it when you lie down. Sit on the end of the blanket, and lie back so that the whole spine and back of the head are supported *(Image 31)*.

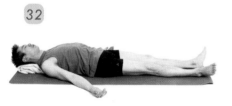

You should feel that the centre of the shoulder blades and the spine are held up slightly into the body by the blanket, allowing the corners of the shoulders to release down more easily *(Image 32)*. Follow the rest of the instructions from *Variation 1*.

WHERE TO PRACTISE

Yoga is best done in a quiet, clean space. However, this isn't always achievable, and it is better to practise somewhere that might at first glance seem a little odd, than not at all.

Here are some suggestions of where you could practise:

In a bathroom

Adho Mukha Svanasana can be done with the hands on the side of a bath
Utthita Hasta Padangusthasana, and Utthita Parsva Hasta Padangusthasana can be done
with the heel resting on a window ledge, or on the top of a cabinet
(one that sits on the floor rather than a wall-mounted cabinet)
Uttanasana with the buttocks resting against a wall can be done leaning on the door
(closed and locked for safety) or against a flat-fronted cabinet

In a bedroom

Adho Mukha Svanasana can be practised with the hands on the edge of a chair
or on a sturdy bedside table
Ardha Uttanasana and preparation for Virabhadrasana 3 can be practised
with the hands on a dressing table or window ledge

In a lounge

Supta Padangusthasana 1 can be practised as a restful posture lying in a doorframe,
with the back of the lifted leg supported against the edge of the door

In a hallway

Parsvottanasana can be practised in a narrow hallway,
as can standing postures practised with the back against a wall

EQUIPMENT THAT YOU MAY NEED FOR YOUR PRACTICE

Some of the sequences use chairs, ledges or walls for support. You may also need
a belt of some sort – a yoga belt is best, as it can be adjusted, but if you don't have one a
dressing-gown belt, if necessary tied to form a loop, is fine. For
supporting parts of the body in seated postures you may
need a few yoga blocks, or folded towels or blankets, or
a few firm cushions. Don't worry about having the 'right'
equipment – use what you can find.

A yoga mat will stop you slipping when you're doing
standing postures, but all the seated postures can be done without one.
Seated postures can be done on a towel or blanket for comfort.

33

Short Programmes
10 - 15 minutes

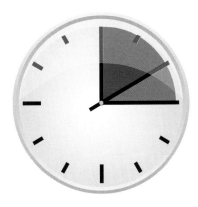

S1 | SHORT PROGRAMME 1

A short sequence to lengthen the spine, gently stretch out the abdomen, strengthen and tone the legs and arms, and mobilise the shoulders, ankles and hip joints

YOU WILL NEED:
- A wall or ledge which is roughly the height of your hips
- A chair or ledge which is roughly knee height

Tadasana with Urdhva Hastasana and Urdhva Baddhanguliyasana

Mountain posture, or standing straight, with arm variations (upward hand pose and upward bound fingers pose)

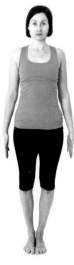

S1.01

Stand with the feet together – or, if they will not come together, as close as they will go *(S1.01)*. Lift the muscles of the thighs. To do this, lift your toes off the floor. Feel the front thighs and kneecaps lift. Keep these actions as you stretch the toes back down to the floor.

Take the weight into the heels, and move the tailbone into the body. Feel the abdomen and spine lift. Take the corners of the shoulders back, and release the muscles of the shoulders away from the ears. Have the hands by the outer thighs, and stretch the fingers to the floor. This is **Tadasana,** or **Samasthiti.**

Arm Variations

Urdhva Hastasana

Have a yoga belt with the loop shoulder-width wide, or a dressing gown belt, knotted *(S1.02)*.

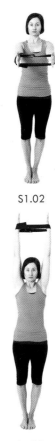

- Put the belt loop around your wrists. Stretch your arms out in front of you, with the palms facing each other. Keep the shoulders away from the ears and the tailbone moving into the body. Reach your hands to the ceiling *(S1.03)*. If this is too painful in the shoulders, loosen the belt so that the hands are wider apart.
- Keep the shoulder muscles extending down, away from the ears. Keep the tailbone in as you reach the hands up. If the shoulders start to hunch or the abdomen swings forward, don't take the hands so high. This applies to all the arm variations. It is more important to keep the correct actions than it is to have the arms back by the ears.
- Keep the weight in the heels, and the thigh muscles lifting throughout.
- Release the hands down.

S1.02

S1.03

Urdhva Baddhanguliyasana

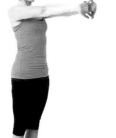

- Interlace your fingers together, turn the palms away from you, press the fingers into the backs of the hands, and straighten the arms *(S1.04)*. Slowly take the hands towards the ceiling *(S1.05)*. Keep the shoulders away from the ears, and the tailbone moving into the body *(S1.06)*. Keep the weight in the heels, and the thigh muscles lifting throughout.
- Release the hands down, and change the interlacing of the fingers, so that the other thumb is on top. Repeat.

S1.04

S1

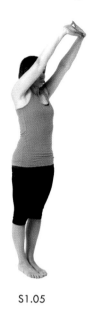

FOCUS ON: Keeping the shoulder muscles drawing away from the ears

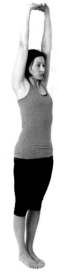

S1.05   S1.06

Ardha Uttanasana

Half intense stretch pose,
or half standing forward bending posture

If you have a flexible lumbar there will be a tendency for it to drop in this posture. To avoid this, hold your abdomen up to your spine, away from the floor.

- Place the hands on a flat surface, at hip height. Walk back until the legs are vertical, with the hips above the heels, and the arms and back straight, in one horizontal line.

- Place the feet hip bone width apart, with the centre lines of the feet parallel.

- Lift the front thigh muscles and reach the very top of your thighs back.

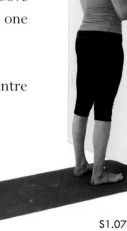

S1.07

- Move the shoulders away from the ears. Feel that the abdomen, spine and side trunk are all elongated by the action of the arms and legs.

- Bend the knees, look forward and step forward to come up.

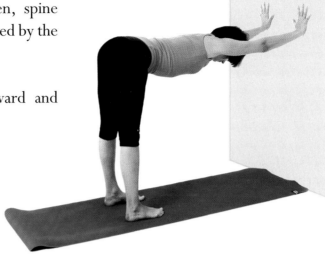

S1.08

Adho Mukha Svanasana

Downward facing dog,
with the hands on a raised support

If you are using a chair and the whole hand can't fit on the seat without the hands being too close, then have just the base of the hands in contact with the chair and stretch the fingers away.

- Place the hands on a flat surface, roughly as high as your knees. Have the hands shoulder width apart. Walk your feet back so that they are behind the line of the hips.
- Have your feet hip bone width apart, with the centre lines of the feet pointing directly forward.
- The legs and arms are straight *(S1.11)*.
- Lift the muscles of your front thighs up and press them back, away from your

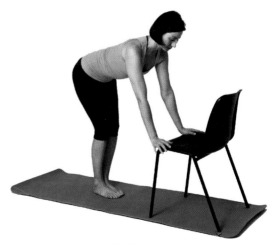

S1.09

S1

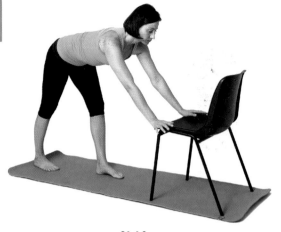

S1.10

hands. To do this, lift your toes; feel your thighs lift. Keep this action on the thighs as you lengthen the toes back down.

•   Let the head and neck hang down.

•   To release, bend the knees, look forward and step forward to come up to a standing position.

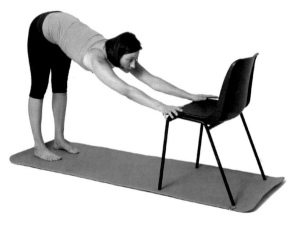

S1.11

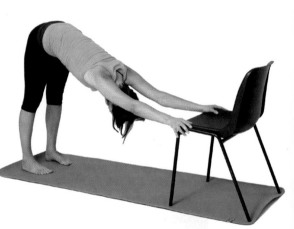

S1.12

Savasana

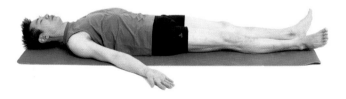

S1.13

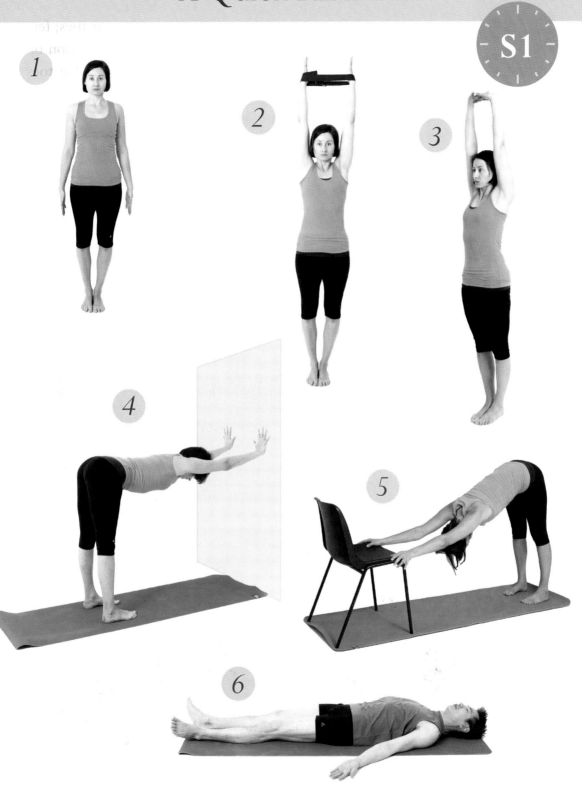

S1

S2 SHORT PROGRAMME 2

*A short sequence to lengthen and mobilise the spine,
strengthen and stretch the legs, and warm up and open
the shoulders and hip joints*

YOU WILL NEED:
- A chair or ledge which is roughly knee height
- A ledge or piece of furniture to rest one foot on – the height you need will
  depend on your flexibility, so you may need to try a few things before
  you find the right height support

YOU MAY NEED:
- Two yoga bricks, or a chair or stool

Adho Mukha Svanasana

*Downward facing dog,
with the hands on a raised support*

- Place the hands on a flat surface, roughly knee height. Spread the hands well.
  Have the hands shoulder width apart. Walk your feet back so that they are

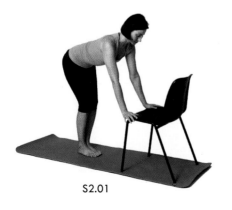

S2.01

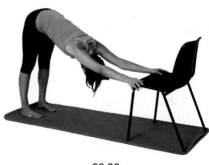

S2.02

behind the line of the hips. Have your feet hip bone width apart, with the centre lines of the feet pointing directly forward. The legs and arms are straight.

- Lift the front thigh muscles up and press them back, away from your hands. Release the shoulder muscles away from the ears. Let the head and neck hang down.
- To release, look forward, bend the knees and step forward to come to standing.

Utthita Hasta Padangusthasana

Extended hand to toe posture,
or standing with one foot raised

When doing this for the first time, spend a little time gauging the right height. The foot should be as high up as you can comfortably take it, but you should be able to keep both legs straight, and the back upright. If you can't, you need to use a slightly lower support for the foot.

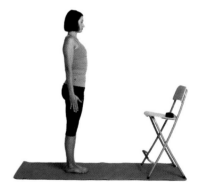

S2.03

- Stand in Tadasana.
- Lift the muscles of the thighs. Take the weight into the heels. Move the tailbone into the body; feel the abdomen and spine lift.
- Bend the right leg, raise the foot and place the back of the heel on your support. Straighten the leg *(S2.06)*. Press the ball of the foot away.
- Keep the standing leg straight, with the thigh well lifted. Stretch the arms up to the ceiling into Urdhva Hastasana, but keep the shoulders

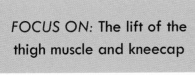

FOCUS ON: The lift of the thigh muscle and kneecap

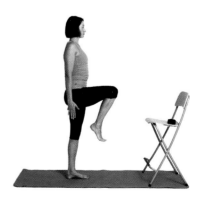

S2.04

S2

releasing down. Lift the chest bone up *(S2.07)*.
- Release the lifted leg down, come back to Tadasana, then change sides.

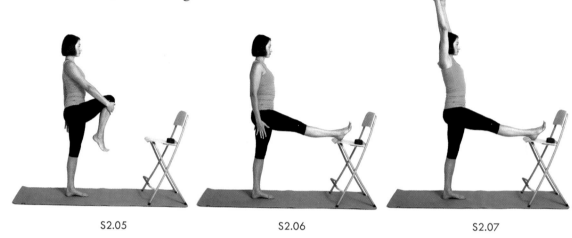

S2.05   S2.06   S2.07

Prasarita Padottanasana, going forward

Wide-legged intense stretch posture, or wide-legged standing forward bend

The height of the support needed in this posture depends on flexibility, but the important action to learn is the extension of the spine.
If your back rounds to the ceiling rather than extending in this posture try taking more support under the hands.

- Stand in Tadasana, on the back of the wide edge of your mat. Step the feet wide apart. Lift the thigh muscles and knee caps strongly up. Keep the tailbone in.
- Take the fingertips onto the hips and extend your chest bone forward, hinging from your hips *(S2.09)*. Extend the front body forward as much as you can, then take the hands down directly under the

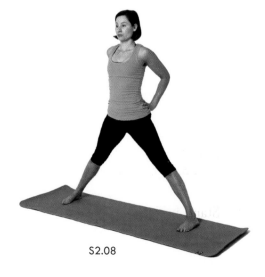

S2.08

shoulders. Use a support if needed. Look forward, and lengthen the chest bone forward to the chin. Keep the shoulder muscles away from the ears.

- To come out of this posture, lift your thigh muscles and your abdomen strongly, take your finger tips to your hips, and reach your chest bone forward then up to come back to a standing position.

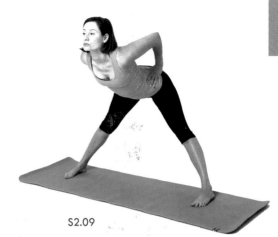

S2.09

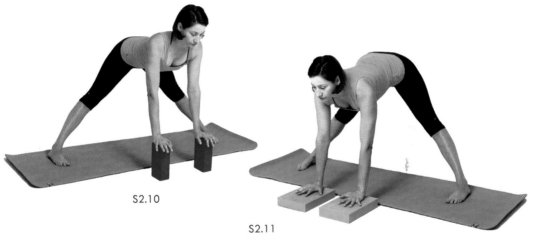

S2.10

S2.11

Uttanasana, going forward

Intense stretch pose,
or forward bend

As with the previous posture, you might need some support under the hands in this posture. Have a few yoga blocks ready nearby. If you are very stiff, you might find a stool or chair is a better height for you.

- Stand in Tadasana with your feet together.
- Keep the legs straight, and lift the muscles of your thighs and your kneecaps up.

S2

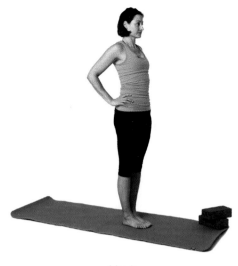

S2.12

• Take your fingertips to your hips and lift your chest bone up, keeping the shoulders away from the ears *(S2.12)*. Hinging from the hips, reach your chest bone forward. Take your hands to your support *(S2.13)*. With straight arms, draw your chest bone forward more. Keep lifting the thigh muscles.

• To come up, lift the muscles of your front thighs further up. Hold your abdomen to your spine. Extend the chest bone forward to come back to a standing position.

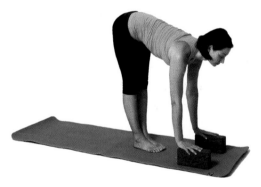

S2.13

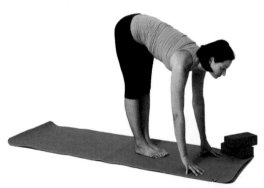

S2.14

Savasana

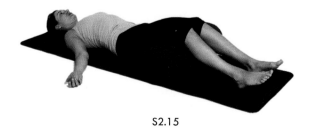

S2.15

S2

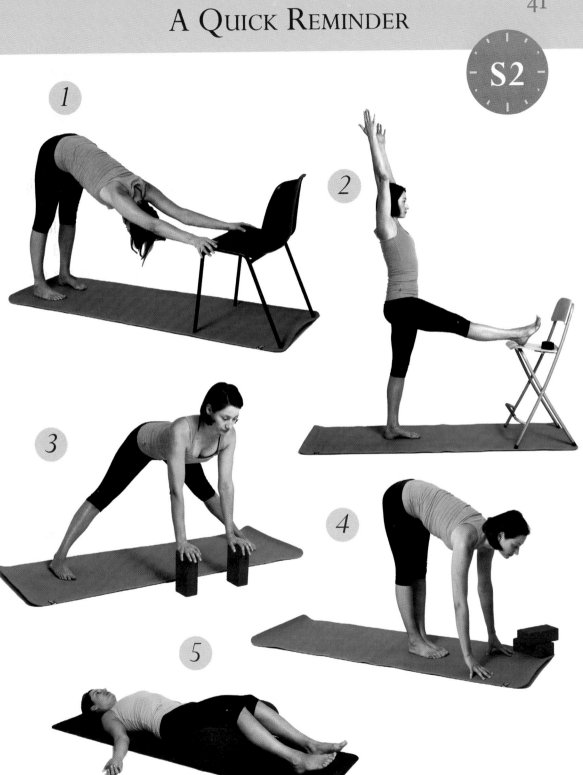

S3 | SHORT PROGRAMME 3

A short sequence to open the hips, mobilise the ankles and shoulders, create length in the spine and abdomen, and open the chest

YOU WILL NEED:
- Cushions, yoga blocks or folded towels
- A belt

Baddha Konasana

Bound angle pose,
or sitting with the soles of the feet together

In this posture, the knees should be in line with or slightly lower than the hips, so that the legs can release down, and the spine can lift up. If your knees are higher than the line of the hips, sit up on a support, until the knees come level with the hips. If this means you need to sit up very high, take some padding under your heels (S3.04), which will encourage the lift of the front body.

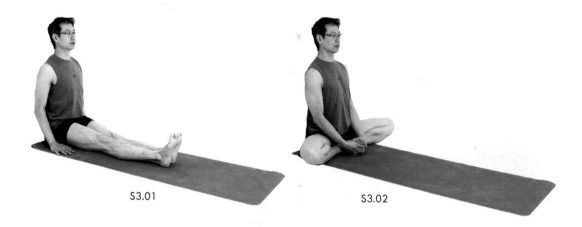

S3.01   S3.02

If you have knee problems, take some support in the back of the knees, and hold it in place as you open the knees wide, as shown in images S3.03 and S3.04.

- Sit with your legs straight out in front of you *(S3.01)*, and your back upright. This is **Dandasana**. Bend the legs, one at a time, taking the knees out wide. Bring the feet in to the centre line of the body, close to but not touching the pelvis. Have the soles of the feet together. Release the knees down to the floor.
- Hold the feet around the toes, or hold the ankles. Lift the sides of the body up. Separate the collar bones, and release the shoulders away from the ears.

Alternative Restful Variation

- If you find it tiring to sit up in this position, you can try a more restful, supported version, with your back against a wall.
- Sit with your back to a wall. Lean forward, and move the buttocks back so that they touch the wall. Place a thin cushion or a flat yoga block behind your lower spine, and sit back. Feel that now the spine can move in, and the front body can lift up.
- Lift the chest bone. Feel the abdomen also lift, and move back gently to the spine. Release the shoulders away from the ears.
- Rest the back of the hands on the thighs.

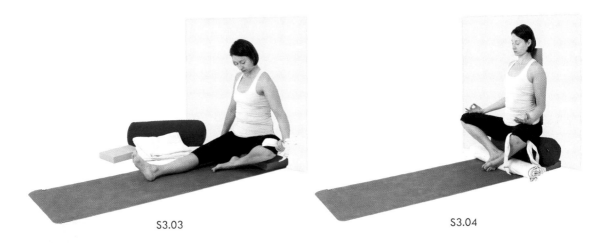

S3.03   S3.04

S3

Virasana,
with the hands clasped behind the back

Virasana is named after a sage
A kneeling position

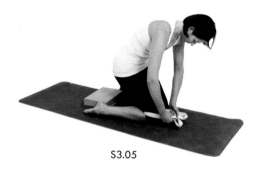

S3.05

If you have knee problems, make sure you sit on enough support to ensure that there is no discomfort in the knees. Also, place support in the back of the knee, such as a yoga belt or a sock, as shown in S3.05, S3.06 and S3.07. If the ankles are very uncomfortable, have some padding under the top of the ankles, as shown on page 15, Image 3.

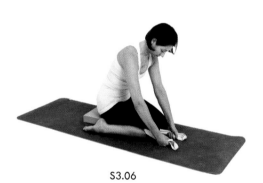

S3.06

• Kneel up. Take the knees together, to touch. Have the top of the feet on the floor, and the feet just wider than your hips.

• Take your thumbs into the backs of the knee joints, and ease the calf muscle gently toward the ankles, and out to the sides. As you do this, sit down in between your feet.

• If the buttocks are not touching the floor between the feet, place some support under the buttock bones. Feel that you are sitting with the spine upright. Move your abdomen back onto your spine. Lift your chest bone up.

• Stretch both arms back. Clasp the hands, and draw the hands back away from the buttocks, and down to the floor *(S3.08)*. Keep the abdomen drawn back to the spine.

• Release, and change the clasp of the hands, so that the other thumb is on top. Repeat.

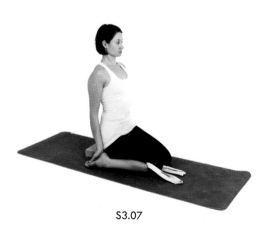

S3.07

FOCUS ON: The lift
of the front body

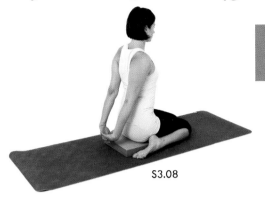

S3.08

Swastikasana

Sitting cross-legged, with the back upright

Your knees should be level with or slightly lower then your hips in this posture, to encourage the lift of the spine. If your knees are higher than your hips, sit up on a firm cushion or support, until the knees come level with the hips. Have the support just under the buttock bones, not under the thighs. Also, if you feel that your lower back is dropping, sit up on a support.

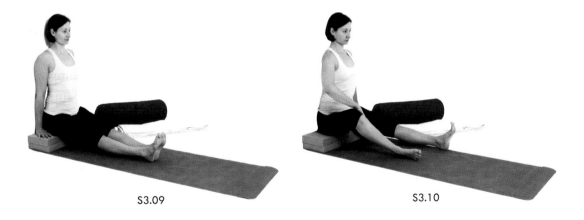

S3.09   S3.10

- Sit with the legs straight out in front of you. Cross the right shin in front of the left, so that the feet are more or less in line with the knees. Have a space between the legs and the pelvis (*S3.11*).
- Feel that you are sitting right on the top of the buttock bones. Place the fingertips down on either side of the hips. Press the fingertips down, and lift

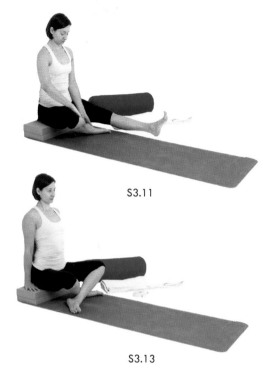

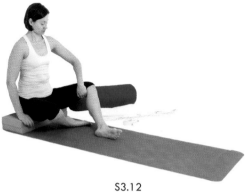

S3.11

S3.12

S3.13

the chest bone and the sides of the body up *(S3.13)*. Release the muscles of the shoulders away from the ears.

• Release, and change the cross of the legs. Sit for even lengths of time on each side.

Alternative Restful Variation

• To make this posture more restful, sit with your back against a wall, as you did in Baddha Konasana, shown at the beginning of this programme. Place a thin cushion or folded blanket behind the spine to encourage the lift of the front body. Let the shoulder muscles release down, away from the ears.

• Remember to change the cross of your legs. Try to sit for even lengths of time on each side, to balance the body.

Savasana

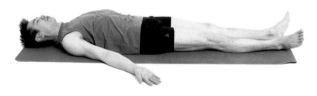

S3.14

S3

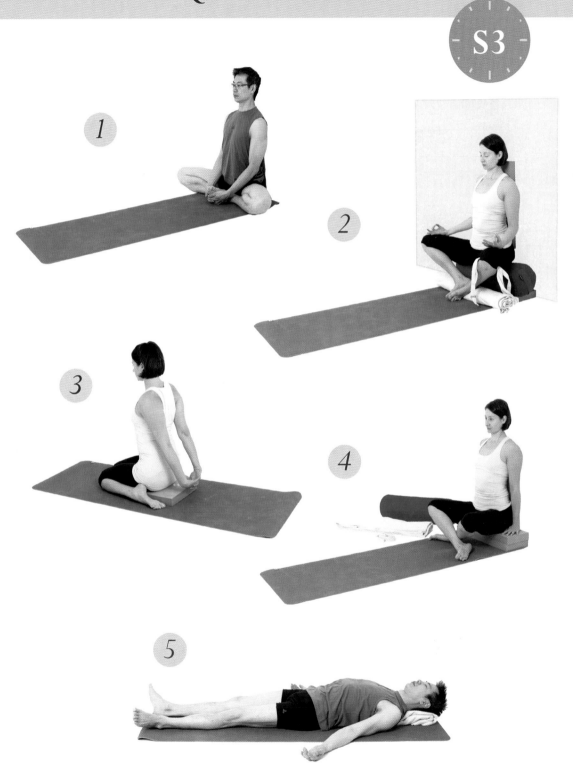

1

2

3

4

5

S4   SHORT PROGRAMME 4

A short sequence to improve the circulation in the feet and legs, lengthen the spine, stretch and tone the legs and mobilise the ankles and hips

YOU WILL NEED:
- A chair or stool which is roughly knee height
- A belt

YOU MAY NEED:
- Yoga blocks or bricks

Tadasana with Urdhva Hastasana and Urdhva Baddhanguliyasana

Mountain posture, or standing straight, with arm variations (upward hand pose and upward bound fingers pose)

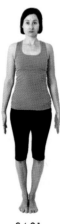

S4.01

• Stand in Tadasana. Lift the kneecaps and front thigh muscles. Take the weight back into the heels, and lengthen the toes along the floor.

• Move the tailbone into the body: feel the abdomen and front spine lift up. Take the corners of the shoulders back, and release the muscles of the shoulders away from the ears. Have the hands by the outer thighs, and stretch the fingers to the floor.

Arm Variations

Urdhva Hastasana

Have a belt with the loop shoulder width.

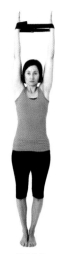

S4.02

- Put the belt around your wrists. Stretch your arms out in front of you, with the palms facing each other. Reach your hands to the ceiling and release your shoulders away from the ears. Keep the weight in the heels, and the thigh muscles lifting throughout *(S4.02)*.

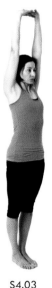

Urdhva Baddhanguliyasana

- Interlace your fingers together, turn the palms away from you, press the fingers into the backs of the hands, and straighten the arms. Slowly take the hands towards the ceiling. Draw the shoulder muscles down. Move the tailbone into the body *(S4.03)*.
- Release the hands down. Change the interlacing of the fingers, so that the other thumb is on top, and repeat.

S4.03

Adho Mukha Svanasana

Downward facing dog, with the hands on a raised support

- Come to Adho Mukha Svanasana with your hands on a chair *(S4.04)*.
- Lift the muscles of your front thighs up and press them back, away from your hands.
- Reach the heel bones down.

S4

- Let the head and neck hang down, and extend the muscles of the shoulders away from the ears *(S4.05)*.

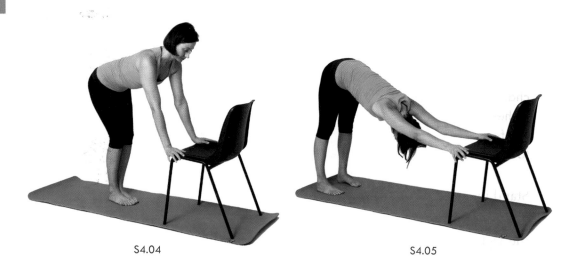

S4.04   S4.05

Preparation for Parsvottanasana

Forward spine extension, with the hands supported

- Be in Adho Mukha Svanasana (downward dog) with your hands on the chair. Feel that the shoulders are releasing away from the ears, the thigh muscles are well lifted, and the hips are level.

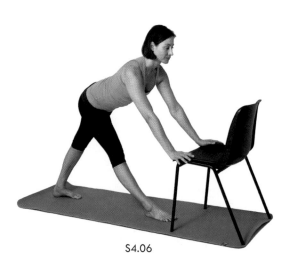

S4.06

- Turn the left toes out slightly, then step the right foot forward. Straighten both legs. Reach the back hip forward and the front hip back, so that the hips are level – remember how they felt level in downward dog, and try to recreate that feeling. Look forward, and extend your chest body forward.
- To release, bend the front leg and come back to downward dog. Change sides.

Parsvottanasana, extending forward

Intense stretch posture to the side,
or a standing extension for the spine

If you found using the chair in the last posture was challenging enough, use the chair again for this variation of the posture, which is coming into it from Tadasana rather than Adho Mukha Svanasana (downward dog). If you felt that it was quite comfortable, have yoga bricks for your hands instead. Place the chair or the bricks towards the front (narrow) edge of your mat.

- Stand in Tadasana at the back of your mat.
- Turn the left toes out slightly, then step the right foot forward about a metre, so that it is centrally placed between your supports *(S4.08)*. Reach the back hip forward and the front hip back, so that the hips are level.
- Take the fingertips to your hips. Keep your thigh muscles well lifted. Reach your chest bone up, then hinge from the hips to extend the chest forward *(S4.09)*. Take

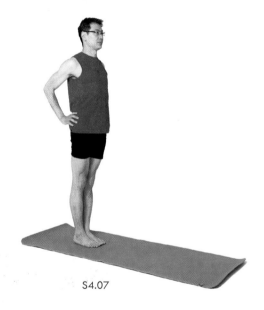

S4.07

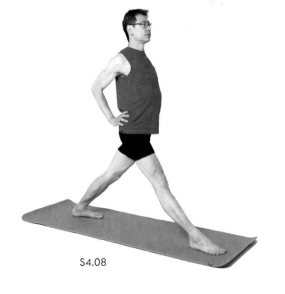

S4.08

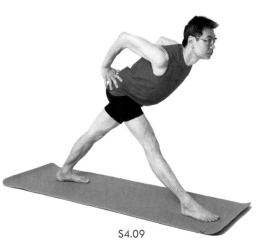

S4.09

S4

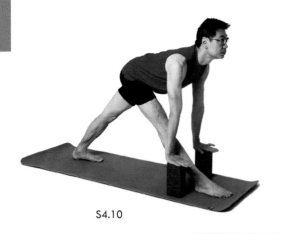

S4.10

your hands onto your support *(S4.10)*. Keep the muscles of the shoulders away from the ears.

• To release, keep the thigh muscles well lifted. Take your fingertips to your hips, and extend the chest bone forward then up to come back to standing. Bend the front leg and step forward. Come back to Tadasana at the back of your mat, and change sides.

> FOCUS ON: The
> alignment of the hips

Savasana

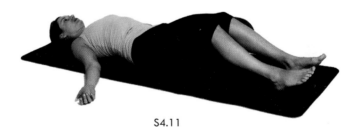

S4.11

S4

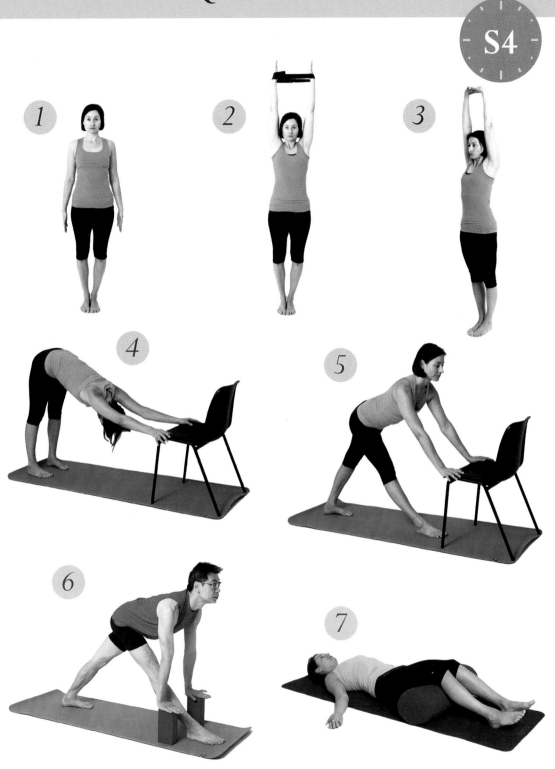

S5 | SHORT PROGRAMME 5

*A short sequence to strengthen the legs, open the hips
and create length in the spine and abdomen*

YOU WILL NEED:
• A wall or vertical support

YOU MAY NEED:
• Cushions or folded towels

Tadasana with Urdhva Baddhanguliyasana and Paschima Namaskarasana

*Mountain pose, with arm variations
(upward bound fingers pose and reverse prayer position)*

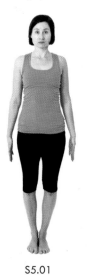

• Stand in Tadasana. Lift the front thigh muscles and kneecaps, and take the weight into the heels.

• Move the tailbone into the body. Take the corners of the shoulders back, and release the muscles of the shoulders away from the ears. Have the hands by the outer thighs, and stretch the fingers to the floor.

S5.01

Arm Variations

Urdhva Baddhanguliyasana

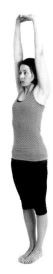

- Take the arms up into Urdhva Baddhan-guliyasana. Reach the thumb side of the hands up further, so that the palms face directly up. Keep the shoulders away from the ears, and the abdomen moving back to the spine. Grip the outer heels in. At the same time, press down into the inner edge of the ball of the foot. Feel that when you get both actions happening together, the central arch of the foot lifts up.
- Release, and change the cross of the fingers. Repeat on the other side.

S5.02

Preparation for Paschima Namaskarasana

- Maintaining the work in the legs and feet, clasp the elbows behind your back. Draw the corners of the elbows slightly away from the buttocks, and down to the floor. Draw the corners of the shoulders back, so that the chest lifts and opens. The back of the head, the back of the sacrum and the heels should be in

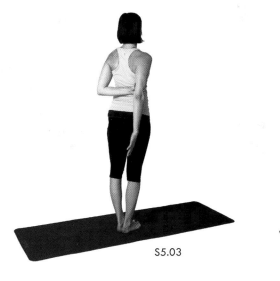

S5.03

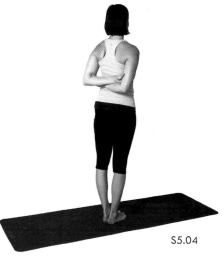

S5.04

one line.
- Release, change the cross of the arms and repeat.

Paschima Namaskarasana

- Bring the palms together behind your back with the fingers pointing down *(S5.05)*. Turn the fingers inward then upwards, so that the fingertips reach to the neck *(S5.07)*. Move the hands up until they sit between the shoulder blades. If they don't come that high, have them wherever is possible. Stretch the fingers to your neck and press the palms together. Take the corners of the shoulders back, and lift the chest bone up *(S5.08)*.

- Release, and stretch the arms out to the sides. Don't shake the hands – the wrists need to be treated gently. Turn the palms up, and stretch the fingers away. Turn the palms back. Finally, release the arms down.

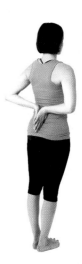

Pic. S5.05

If Paschima Namaskarasana is too strong on the wrists or shoulders, continue to work into the preparatory posture.

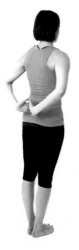

Pic. S5.06

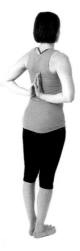

Pic. S5.07

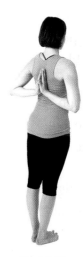

Pic. S5.08

Virabhadrasana 2

Warrior 2 pose – standing with one leg bent and one straight

Using the wall for this posture is more restful, but it also allows you to learn the alignment better. The next time you practise, try moving away from the wall. If you struggle to achieve the correct alignment, go back to the wall.

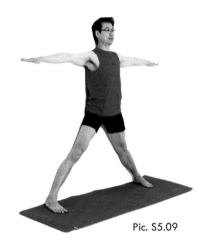

Pic. S5.09

- Stand in Tadasana, with your back against a wall.

- Step the legs wide apart, and have the feet pointing forward. At the same time, stretch your arms out at shoulder height.

- Turn your left toes in a little, so your left foot is angled inward, and turn your right leg fully out, so that your right foot is parallel to the wall *(S5.10)*. Rest your right outer hip against the wall, and move your tailbone away from the wall. Look along your right fingers, and bend your right leg so that it comes as close to a right angle as possible. The knee should be above the ankle *(S5.11)*.

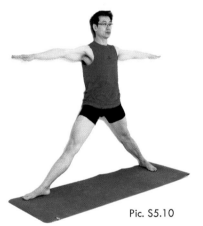

Pic. S5.10

- Open the right knee to the wall, and move the tailbone away from the wall. Release the shoulders away from the ears.

- Straighten the right leg, turn the toes forward, and change sides.

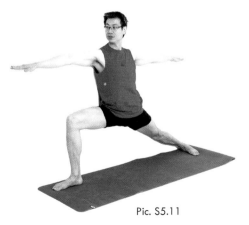

Pic. S5.11

Supta Baddha Konasana

S5

Supine bound angle pose, with or without arm variations

- Lie down, with the knees bent and the soles of the feet flat on the floor. Take the soles of the feet together, so the knees release out and down. Reach the shoulder muscles away from the ears. Lengthen the tailbone and buttocks towards the heels.

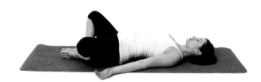

Pic. S5.12

Arm Variations

Variation 1

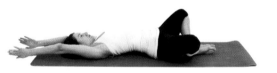

Pic. S5.13

- Extend your hands back to the floor behind your head. Have the palms facing each other, and the hands shoulder width apart. If there is stiffness in the shoulders, take the hands a little wider, and place some support underneath them. Draw the shoulders away from the ears.
- Lengthen the tailbone to the heels, and draw the outer knees towards the floor.

Variation 2

- Clasp the elbows and take them to the floor behind your head. Press the heels lightly together, and extend the inner thighs away, so the outer knees move down.
- Keep the shoulders releasing away from the ears, and the elbows extending away from the shoulders.
- Change the cross of the arms, and repeat.

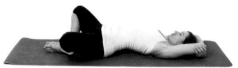

Pic. S5.14

Variation 3

S5

- Interlace the fingers, turn the palms away, and take the hands to the floor behind your head. Lengthen the flesh of your buttocks to your heels, and extend the inner thighs away.

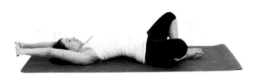
Pic. S5.15

- Press the fingers into the backs of the hands to open the palms, and move the shoulders away from the ears.
- Change the interlacing of the fingers, and repeat.
- To come up, bend your knees by sliding the feet towards you, one at a time. Bend the arms so the hands come to rest on your body. Roll carefully on to your right side, keeping the knees bent. Let the top arm fall in front of the chest, so that the shoulders and hips are stacked on top of each other. Support the head with the lower arm, or a block or blanket. Press yourself up to sitting from your side, so that you don't disturb your back as you come up.

Savasana

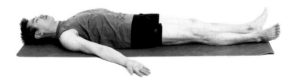
Pic. S5.16

A Quick Reminder

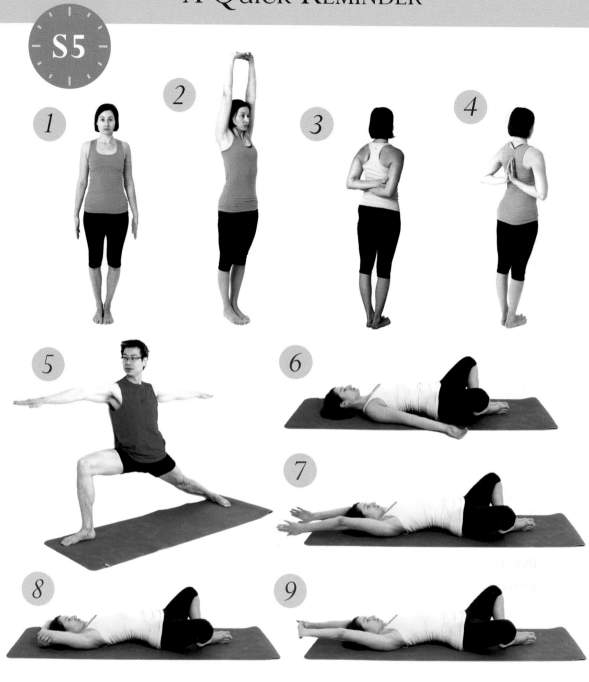

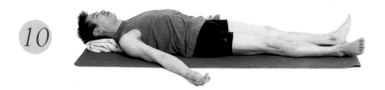

SHORT PROGRAMME 6   S6

A short sequence to strengthen and tone the legs and arms, create length in the spine and mobilise the hips and shoulders

YOU WILL NEED:
- A belt
- A ledge at hip height (or a wall)
- A wall or vertical support

Supta Padangusthasana 1

Supine hand to toe pose, or lying with one leg raised vertically, eventually holding the toe

- Lie down, with your knees bent, and your feet touching a wall. Move the muscles of the shoulders away from the ears, and lengthen the tailbone and buttock flesh to the heels. Feel that the abdomen is releasing down towards the spine.

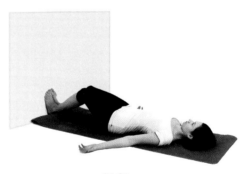

S6.01

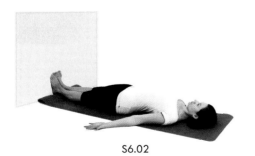

S6.02

- Straighten both legs, pressing yourself away from the wall. Keep the balls of the feet pressing into the wall firmly, so that the legs feel very active. This is Supta Tadasana, with the feet to a wall.

S6

- Bend the right leg and bring the knee towards the chest. Place a belt around the ball of the foot. Then straighten the leg, reaching the foot into the belt towards the ceiling. Hold the belt with both hands, with the hands apart.

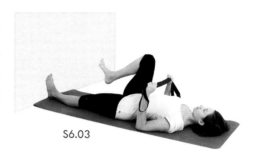

S6.03

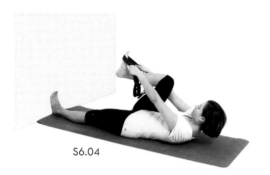

S6.04

- If the foot does not come vertically in line with the hip, take it only as high as it will comfortably come – it is more important to keep the leg straight than to take it closer to the face. Keep reaching the foot into the belt.

- Move the shoulders away from the ears, and separate your collar bones. Press the thigh muscle of the lifted leg away from your face, and lengthen the outer hip away from its own armpit, so the hips are level.

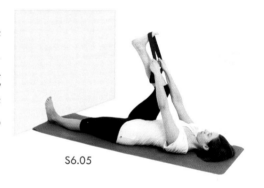

S6.05

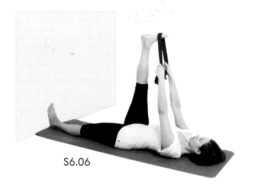

S6.06

- Reach the balls of both feet away from you strongly – press the lower foot into the wall, and the upper foot into the belt.
- Release, and change sides.

FOCUS ON: The action of the ball of the foot on the lifted and lower leg

Preparation for Virabhadrasana 3

Warrior 3

- Start in Ardha Uttanasana, with the hands on a ledge, or on a wall.
- Lift the front thigh muscles and move them back, onto the bones of the thighs. Move the shoulders away from the ears, and take the shoulder blades down to the floor. Hold your abdomen to your spine.

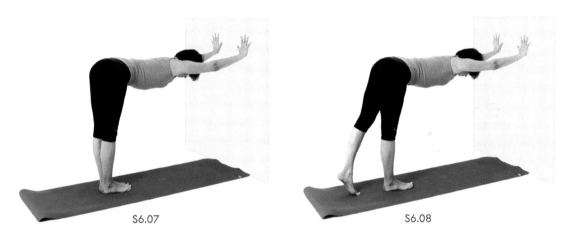

S6.07   S6.08

- Take your left toes back, so they rest on the floor behind the line of your hip. Keep your left hip down, in line with your right.
- Keep your toes pointing down to the floor, and lift your left thigh, until the foot is in line with the hip. If either leg bends, don't take the lifted leg so high – it is more important that the legs are straight. Reach into the ball of the lifted foot.

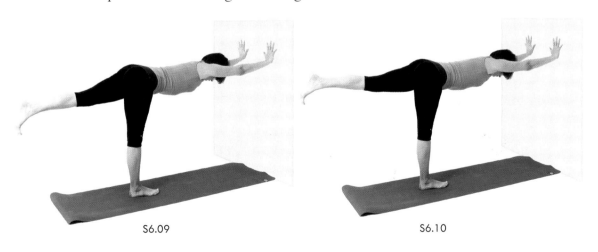

S6.09   S6.10

S6

Keep the thigh of the standing leg lifted. Lengthen the outer hip of the standing leg away from its own armpit, so there is even length on both sides of the body.
• Release the leg back down, and bring the feet together. Repeat on the other side.

Viparita Karani

Inverted action pose, or lying with the legs up the wall

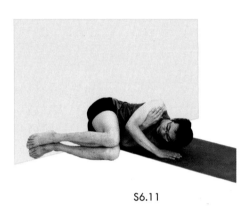

S6.11

• Lie on your side, with your buttocks close to a wall, and your knees bent towards your chest *(S6.11)*. Roll on to your back and straighten the legs up the wall, resting the backs of your heels on the wall. If your legs won't straighten in this position, move away from the wall a little, until they do. Move the muscles of the shoulders away from the ears.

Variations

Variation 1

• Have the feet together, or as close as they will go. Reach the balls of the feet firmly to the ceiling – as if you were pushing the ceiling away. Feel that the

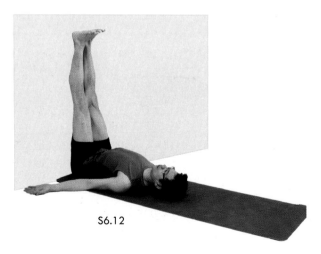

S6.12

muscles of the front thighs and the bones of the thighs are moving down, towards the hips.
• Press the front thighs towards the wall, so that they hold the bones of the thighs. Have the backs of the hands on the floor, with the arms a small distance away from the sides of the trunk.

S6

Variation 2

- Keep the feet reaching away, but take the legs wide. The centre of the backs of the heels should remain in contact with the wall, so the feet don't turn down, or curl to the ceiling – they stay extending away, in line with the legs *(S6.13)*. Move the shoulders away from the ears more, then take your hands over your head towards the floor, keeping the wrists in line with the shoulders *(S6.14)*.
- If the hands don't easily come down to the floor, take them wider, and if they still don't come down, rest them on a cushion or some support. Press the top of your thighs to the wall and reach the fingers away, but keep the shoulders away from the ears. Feel that the sides of the body lengthen.

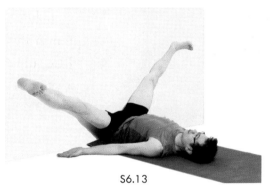

S6.13

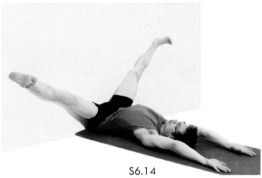

S6.14

- To come down, release the arms down first. Take the legs together again up the wall, then bend the legs and slide the feet towards your buttocks. Roll on to your side, then press yourself up to sitting.

A Resting Variation

- Before you go up into Viparita Karani, take a belt and loop it around your thighs. If you have two belts, place the second belt around your lower legs.

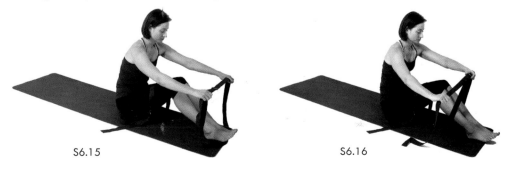

S6.15   S6.16

S6

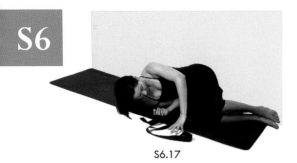

S6.17

- Then roll onto your back and take your legs up the wall as normal.
- From here, bend your knees a little, tighten the belts to hold your legs together, then straighten the legs. Having the legs fixed in this way will allow the legs to relax fully.

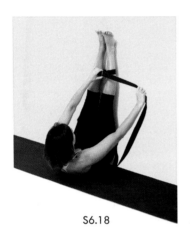

S6.18

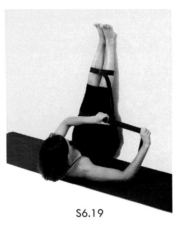

S6.19

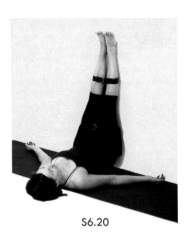

S6.20

BENEFITS:

Viparita Karani

- Revives tired legs
- Gently lengthens the hamstrings
- When done as an active posture, stretches the back and abdomen and opens the chest. When done as a recuperative posture, allows the back and abdomen to lengthen and the chest to open without effort
- Encourages quietness in the mind

Savasana

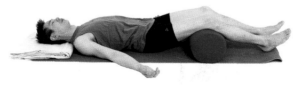

S6.21

S6

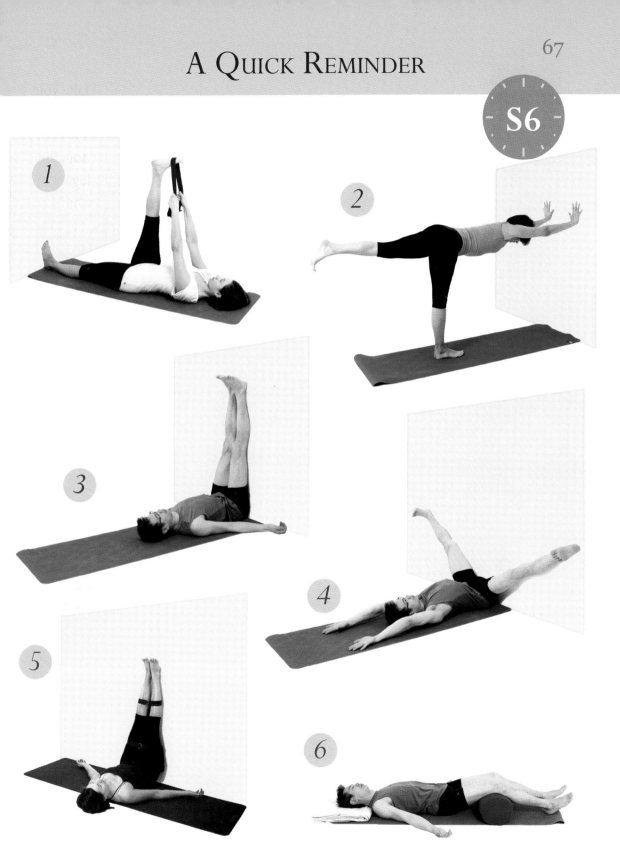

Medium Programmes
20 - 25 minutes

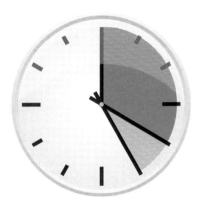

M1 | MEDIUM PROGRAMME 1

*A sequence to strengthen and tone the legs,
lengthen the spine and open the hips and shoulders*

YOU WILL NEED:
- A wall

YOU MAY NEED:
- A belt
- Cushions or a folded towel or blanket
- Blocks or a low stool

Tadasana with Urdhva Baddhanguliyasana and Gomukhasana

*Tadasana with arm variations (backward extension,
upward bound fingers pose and cow face pose)*

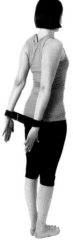

- Stand in Tadasana. Take your thigh muscles up and back, so that you feel that the weight of the body is balanced over the fronts of the heels and the backs of the balls of the feet.

Arm Variations

Variation 1

- Have a belt with the loop shoulder width. Put it around your wrists, behind your back. Have the palms facing each other. Stretch your fingers, and reach the hands away from the buttocks, and down towards the floor. Feel that the shoulders move away from the ears

M1.01

as you extend the fingers away. Extend the arms back and down. Move the tailbone into the body, and lift the chest bone up.

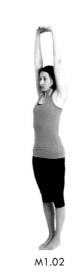

M1

Variation 2

- Interlace your fingers together in front of you, turn the palms away, press the fingers into the backs of the hands, and straighten the arms. Slowly take the arms into Urdhva Baddhanguliyasana. Keep the shoulders away from the ears, and the tailbone moving into the body *(M1.02)*.

M1.02

- Release, change the cross of the fingers, and repeat.

Variation 3

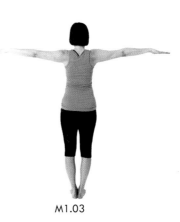

- Bring the arms out wide, in line with the shoulders. Bend your right arm so that your hand is behind your back, in line with the spine *(M1.05)*. Ease the hand as high up the spine as it will go. Draw the corner of the right shoulder back. Take your left hand to the ceiling. Turn the arm so that your palm faces your ear *(M1.06)*, then turn it further, to face back. Keep this turn of the upper arm,

M1.03

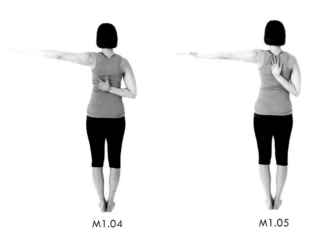

M1.04   M1.05

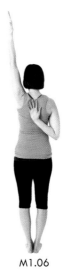

M1.06

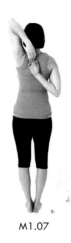

M1.07

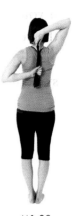

M1.08

so the armpit opens, but stays facing forward *(M1.07)*.

• Bend the elbow, dropping the hand down the back. Catch the hands. If they don't catch, hold a belt in your upper hand, and catch it with the lower hand *(M1.08)*. Ease the fingers closer together. Keep the chest bone lifted, and the corner of the right shoulder back.

• Release and change sides.

Utthita Trikonasana

Extended triangle posture – a standing lateral extension of the spine

The first time you do this, have your back to a wall to aid your alignment. The next time you practise, try being in the centre of the room. If you lose the correct actions, go back to the wall. You can also practise with the back to the wall to make this posture more restful.

• Stand in Tadasana, with your back to the wall. Step the feet about a metre apart, and open your arms wide. Engage your tailbone into the body and lift your thigh muscles up. Reach the shoulders away from the ears.

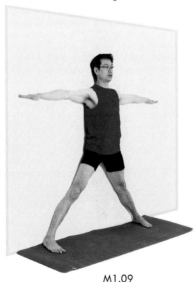

M1.09

• Turn your left toes in a little, so the left foot is angled inward. Turn your right leg fully to the right, so that the outer right thigh is facing the wall and your knee is pointing in the same direction as your toes *(M1.10)*. Rest your right outer hip against the wall. Look at your right big toe.

• Extend your right finger tips as far to the right as you can, then take your hand down onto your shin or ankle. Stretch your left fingers to the ceiling. Move the tailbone in. Rotate your right thigh from the inside to the outside and lift the thigh muscles on both legs *(M1.11)*.

M1

- If you have your balance, turn your abdomen to the ceiling, turn your chest to the ceiling, and finally turn your face to the ceiling.
- To come up, pull your top hand up the ceiling to bring yourself back to a standing position. Turn your toes to face forward, then change sides.

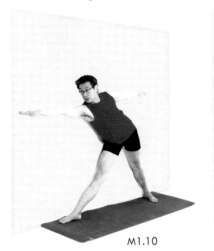

M1.10

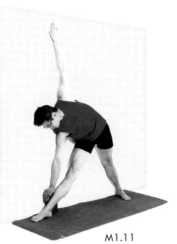

M1.11

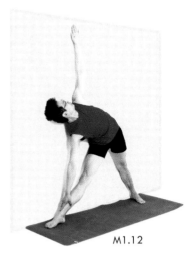

M1.12

Ardha Chandrasana

Half moon posture — standing balancing on one leg

Again, have your back against the wall to begin with, then try to move away from the wall when you have learnt the correct alignment. You can also practise with the back to the wall to make this posture more restful.

You may need a brick or support of some kind for the front hand. Have one ready towards the narrow edge of your mat — you will be going to the right side first.

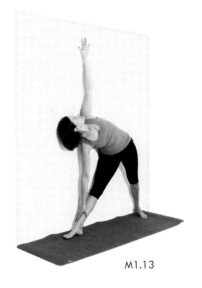

M1.13

- Be in Utthita Trikonasana going to the right *(M1.13)*.
- Look down at your front big toe. Place your left hand on your hip *(M1.14)*. Bend your front leg, reach your right hand forward *(M1.15)* onto the floor or onto your support *(M1.18)*, and hop your back toes in

M1

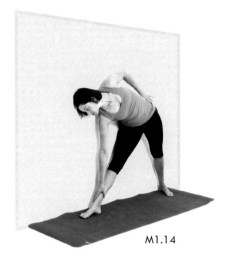

M1.14

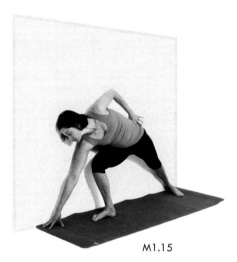

M1.15

a little. From here, straighten your front leg and lift your back leg until the heel comes in line with the hip – or if this is not possible, just as high as it will go *(M1.16)*.

• Lift both thigh muscles. Keep the front thigh rotating from the inside to the outside, so your knee points in the same direction as your toes. Keep your right outer hip on the wall for balance. Stretch your left hand to the ceiling. Move your tailbone in and turn your abdomen and your chest to the ceiling. If you feel you are balanced, turn your face to the ceiling *(M1.17)*.

• To come down, first look down. Place your top hand on your hip, bend your front leg and reach your back leg away until the foot comes to the floor, back in your Utthita Trikonasana position. Come to Utthita Trikonasana, then pull your top hand to the ceiling to lift yourself back to vertical. Turn the feet to face forward, and change sides.

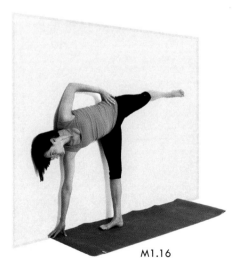

M1.16

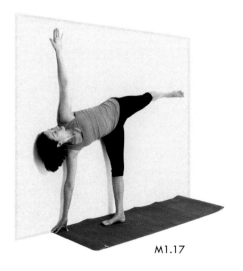

M1.17

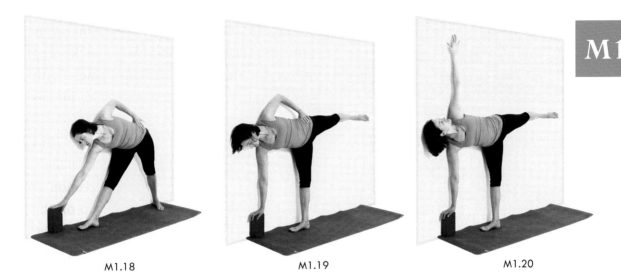

M1

M1.18   M1.19   M1.20

Dandasana with Urdhva Hastasana

Staff pose,
or sitting with the legs straight, with the arms raised

If you find it difficult to sit with the legs straight in this posture, or if your back slumps, sit up on a support — try a yoga block, or a folded towel or blanket.

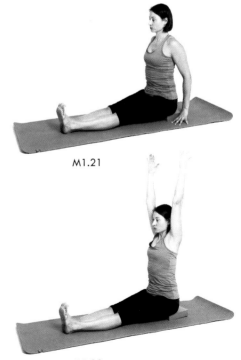

M1.21

- Sit down with the legs extended and the back upright.
- Have the fingertips on the floor either side of the hips, and press the fingertips down to help lift your chest bone up. Extend the balls of the feet away, and release the shoulder muscles away from the ears *(M1.21)*.
- Stretch your arms straight up, but keep the shoulders away from the ears. Reach into the fingers and the wrists, and lift the side body up *(M1.22)*.

M1.22

Janu Sirsasana

M1

*Head to knee posture,
or bending forward, with one leg bent*

If you have a knee problem, take a belt or a sock into the back of the bent knee, as shown in the section on knee problems. If the bent knee doesn't come to the floor in this position, sit up on a support so that the knee can release down to the mat. If you can't easily reach the foot, use a belt — have one ready nearby.

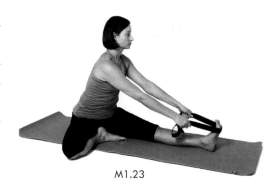

M1.23

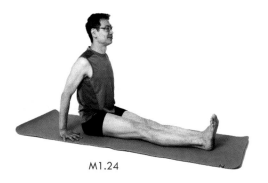

M1.24

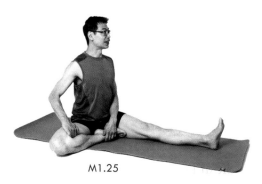

M1.25

- Be in Dandasana. Bend your right knee wide to the side, so that the sole of the foot comes into the inner thigh of the straight leg. Lift the sides of your body up. Lengthen your chest bone forward towards the extended leg. Reach the arms forward, clasp around the edges of the foot, press the foot into the hands, and extend the chest bone forward more *(M1.26)*.

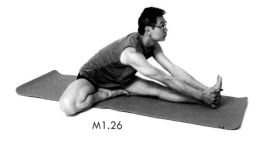

M1.26

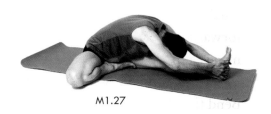

M1.27

- If you can't reach the foot, take a belt around the ball of the foot, and press the foot into the belt to extend the chest forward.
- Keep the shoulders away from the ears. If you are holding the foot, bend the elbows wide, extend the side ribs forward, then rest the head down *(M1.27)*.
- To come up, look up, release the foot or belt, and lift your chest to come back to an upright position. Stretch your legs out in front of you.
- Change sides and repeat.

Triang Mukhaikapada Paschimottanasana

Three-limbed, face to one leg,
intense stretching forward bend posture

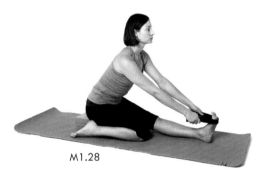

M1.28

If you can't reach the foot in this posture, take a belt around the foot and hold it with both hands. If you can't lift the back up in Dandasana, or if you can't sit with the buttocks on the floor in Virasana, sit up on a support, placing it just underneath the buttock bones.

- Sit in Dandasana.
- Bend the right leg into Virasana. Feel that the hips are level. Draw the right outer hip down and pin the right buttock bone down. If you feel that you're tipping, place a support under the left outer thigh or hip.
- Lift the chest, and extend the sides of the body. Feel that the front body is lifting fully. Reach the arms forward, and hold the outside edges of the foot. Extend the chest forward. Draw the front and back thigh muscles of the extended leg back towards the body, but reach the ball of the foot away.
- Bend the elbows and lift them up a little, to

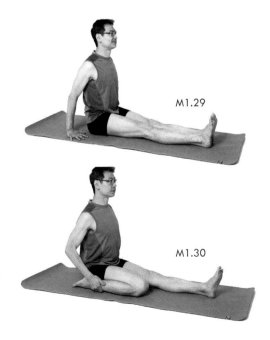

M1.29

M1.30

M1

extend the side ribs forward more, and allow the head to release down.
- To come up, look forward. Release the foot or belt. Extend the chest forward and up to return to an upright position. Stretch both legs out in front of you.
- Change sides.

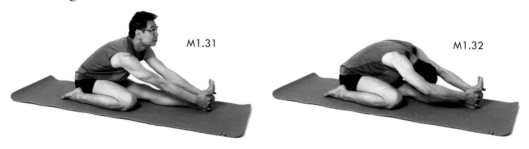

M1.31   M1.32

Supta Baddha Konasana

Supine bound angle posture

- Lie down in Supta Baddha Konasana.
- Extend the inner thighs away to bring the outer knees down. Keep the tailbone flowing to the heels.

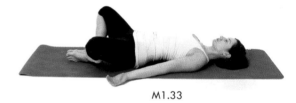

M1.33

Arm Variations

Variation 1

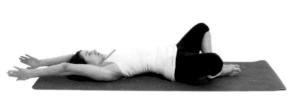

M1.34

- Stretch your fingers to the floor behind your head, with the palms facing each other, shoulder width apart. Keep the shoulders away from the ears. Lengthen the back of the tailbone to the heels.
- Reach your thumbs away more. Feel that this extends the back and side ribs further away from the waist, lengthening the body.

Variation 2

- Clasping your elbows, reach the elbows towards the floor behind your head. Draw the corners of the elbows away from you, but keep the shoulders moving away from the ears. Engage the shoulder blades up towards the chest, and feel the elbows release down more.
- Release, change the cross of the forearms, and repeat on the other side.

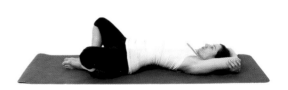

M1.35

Variation 3

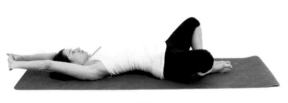

M1.36

- Interlace your fingers together, and take the hands towards the floor behind your head. Draw the pubic bone to the navel, the navel to the chest bone, and the chest bone to the chin.
- Release, change the interlacing of the fingers and repeat.

Savasana

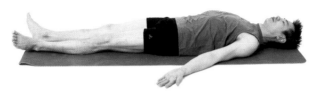

M1.37

A QUICK REMINDER

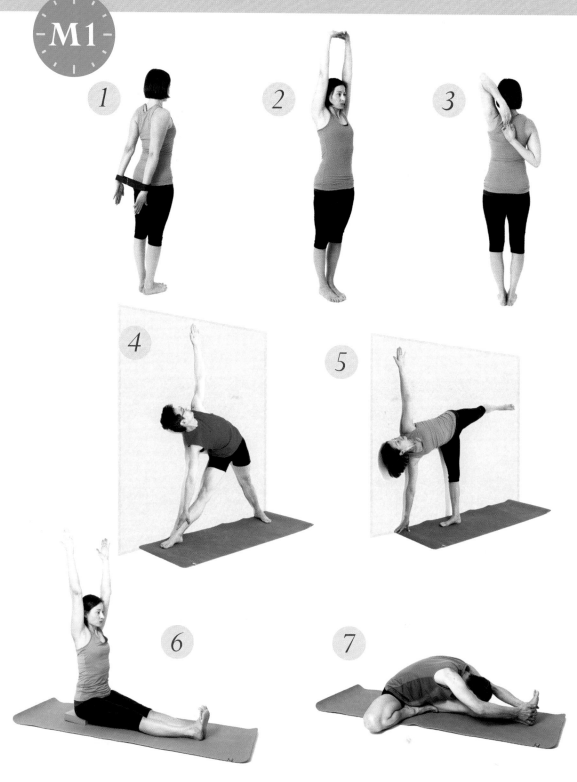

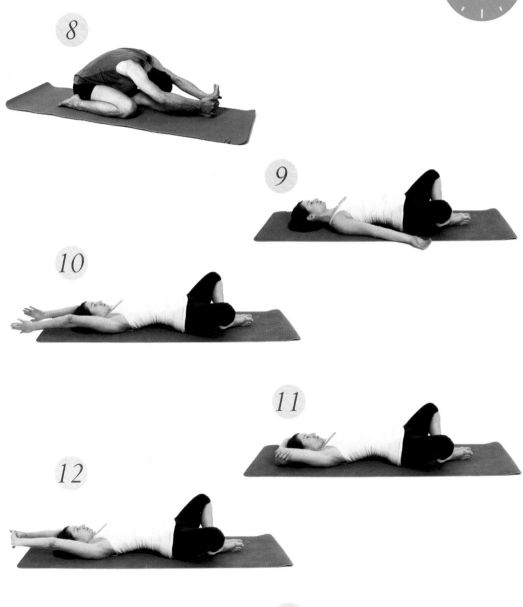

8

9

10

11

12

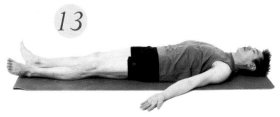

13

M2 | MEDIUM PROGRAMME 2

A sequence to strengthen and tone the legs and buttocks, lengthen the spine and open the hips

YOU WILL NEED:
- A belt
- A wall or vertical support

YOU MAY NEED:
- Cushions or folded towels or blankets

Supta Tadasana

Supine mountain pose, or lying flat

- Lie down in Supta Tadasana.
- Reach the shoulder muscles away from the ears. Lengthen the buttocks and the tailbone towards the heels. Draw the pubic bone to the navel, the navel to the chest bone, and the chest bone to the chin.
- Reach the inner edges of the balls of the feet away from you, so that the balls of the feet broaden and the little toes come slightly back towards your head.

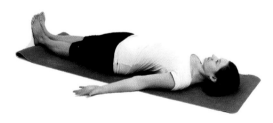

M2.01

Supta Padangusthasana 1 and 2

Supine hand to toe postures
Lying down with leg extensions two ways: vertical and to the side

- Lie down in Supta Tadasana *(M2.01)*.
- Come into Supta Padangusthasana 1 with a belt around the ball of the raised right foot *(M2.02)*.
- Straighten the leg, reaching the ball of the foot away, but resisting this action with the belt so that you pull the thigh bone back down, into the hip socket. Draw the lifted leg towards your face as much as it will go.
- Take the belt into the right hand. Without disturbing your hips or shoulders, open your leg wide to the side. Keep the foot moving up to the line of the shoulder. Bend your right arm and place your elbow on the floor, in line with your shoulder.
- As you take the leg to the side, move the right buttock and the right side of the sacrum to the ceiling, so you don't feel that you're tipping to the lifted leg side. Keep both feet extending away firmly.
- Lift the leg back to centre, and release. Change sides.

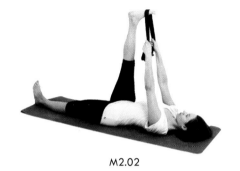

M2.02

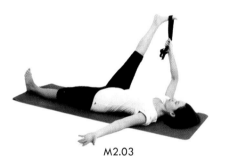

M2.03

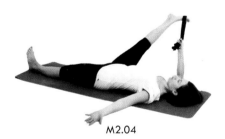

M2.04

BENEFITS:
Supta Padangusthasana 1 and 2
- Strengthens and tones the legs and arms
- Mobilises the hips, sacrum and spine, improving flexibility
- Lengthens the abdomen and spine
- Tones the abdominal, back and buttock muscles
- Opens the pelvis and chest

Vrksasana

M2

Tree posture, or standing balancing with one leg bent

The first time you practise this have your back against a wall, to learn the alignment. After that, you can practise free standing and improve your balance. If you start to lose the alignment, go back to the wall.

If you can't take the foot up into the inner thigh, place the foot on the inner calf of the straight leg instead — don't have the foot against the knee.

- Stand in Tadasana. Lift your right leg, open the knee wide to the right, and take your ankle with your right hand. Lift your foot and place it high up on the centre of the inner left thigh, with the toes pointing down *(M2.07)*. Press the foot into the inner thigh, and grip your left outer thigh towards your foot, so that the foot stays in position.
- Stretch your arms to the ceiling, with the palms facing each other. Keep the shoulders away from the ears, and grip the upper arms in *(M2.09)*.

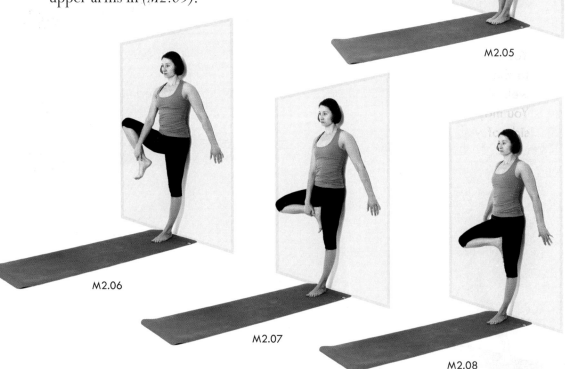

M2.05

M2.06

M2.07

M2.08

- Open the bent knee back to the wall, but move the tailbone and the right buttock forward, so that the hips open.
- Press the foot to the thigh and the thigh to the foot. Move the tailbone in, and lift the chest bone up.
- Release the arms down, then release the foot, and change sides.

FOCUS ON: The action of the bent leg, which opens back, and the buttock, which moves forward

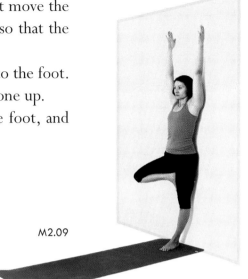

M2.09

M2

Utthita Parsvakonasana

*Extended side angle pose,
or standing lateral extension of the spine*

You can start by practising this against a wall, to improve alignment, and then move to the centre of the room to improve your stamina once the alignment is coming well. You can also practise against a wall to make this posture more restful.
You may need a block for your hand – have one ready towards the right (narrow) side of your mat.

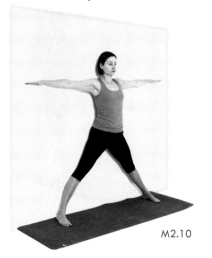

M2.10

- Stand in Tadasana. Step your legs wide apart, and at the same time extend your arms out.

- Turn your right foot and leg fully to the right. Rotate your thigh from the inside to the outside, and rest your outer right hip against the wall. Move the right buttock forward, into the body, so the hips open *(M2.11)*.

M2

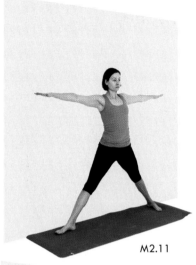

M2.11

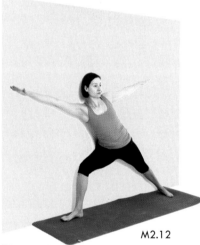

M2.12

• Bend your right leg to a right angle. Keep the knee opening towards the wall, and your tailbone in. Lift the left thigh muscle, and move it back towards the wall, so the hips open strongly *(M2.12)*.

• From here, extend your right fingertips to the right, and reach your right hand onto the outside of your right foot, between the foot and the wall.

• If you can't reach the floor, have a block for the hand. Stretch your left fingers to the ceiling *(M2.13)*. Turn your abdomen and chest to the ceiling, then reach your left fingertips diagonally away from your back foot, until the upper arm almost touches your ear. Look up underneath the upper arm *(M2.14)*.

• To come out of this posture, look forward, pull yourself back to vertical with the upper hand, then turn the feet forward. Change sides.

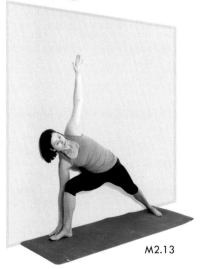

M2.13

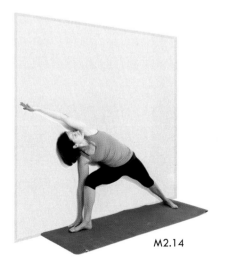

M2.14

Setu Bandha Sarvangasana, with support

Bridge posture, which when done with support is a supine front-opening pose

> If you are fairly stiff in the spine or shoulders, or have back problems, have a low support under the pelvis for this posture, to make the action gentler. If you are quite flexible, have a higher support. To make this posture feel less strong, have the feet hip bone width apart.

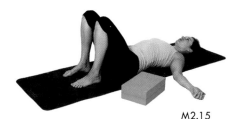

M2.15

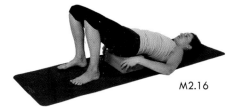

M2.16

- Lie down, with the knees bent. Press the feet down, lift your hips up, and place your support under the sacrum. Move the shoulders firmly away from the ears, then lengthen the flesh of the buttocks to the heels *(M2.16)*.

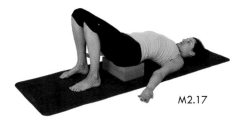

M2.17

- Extend the legs away one at a time. Press the backs of the heels down, and engage the tailbone up into the body. Reach the balls of the feet away. Keep the feet and legs very active: this will prevent any strain in the lower back *(M2.18)*.

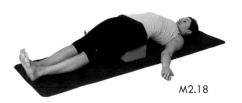

M2.18

- To release, bend your legs, and bring the soles of the feet to the floor. Lift your pelvis *(M2.19)*, remove your support, and pull the tailbone to the heels to lengthen the spine down. Roll to your side to come up.

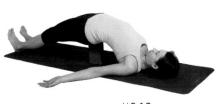

M2.19

M2

Swastikasana, Parsva Swastikasana, then Adho Mukha Swastikasana

Sitting upright with the legs crossed, then turning to the side, then going forward and resting the head

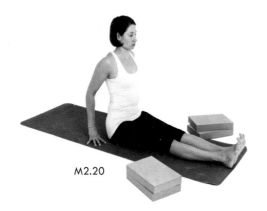

M2.20

The knees should be in line with or lower than the hips in this posture, and the spine should be well lifted. If you find that the legs are lifting or the back dropping, sit up on a support. If the knees, ankles or feet are uncomfortable, have some padding underneath them.

Swastikasana

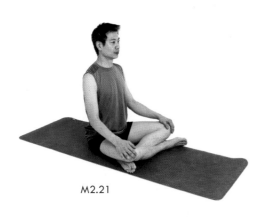

M2.21

• Sit in Dandasana *(M2.20)*. Cross the shins, so that the feet are moved well away from each other, and the knees look forward rather than out to the sides. Have a gap between the pelvis and the floor. Feel that the placement of the legs brings firmness to the hips, and allows the spine to lift.

• Lift the sides of the body up. Lift the sides and back of the neck. Keep the shoulders away from the ears.

• Release the position, stretch out the legs, and then change the cross of the shins. Repeat.

Parsva Swastikasana

- Take your right hand behind you, either onto the floor or onto the edge of your support. Press the hand down to encourage the lift of the spine.
- Take the left hand onto the outer right thigh, close to the knee. Press the hand against the thigh, and resist the leg into the hand. Turn your chest and abdomen to the right, and then turn the head *(M2.22)*.
- Keep the legs releasing down, the spine lifting up, and the corners of the shoulders drawing back.
- Release, and change sides.
- Change the cross of the legs and repeat to both sides.

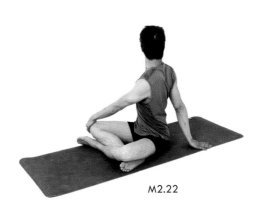

M2.22

Adho Mukha Swastikasana

- Be in Swastikasana. From here, reach the hands forward. Keep the buttock bones pointing down and pinning down, and extend the front of the body forward. When you have lengthened the body well, release the head down. If it doesn't come to the floor, place a support underneath the forehead *(M2.24)*. Rest the head and the neck.
- Release, change the cross of the legs, and repeat.

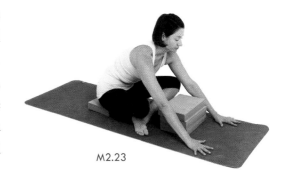

M2.23

M2

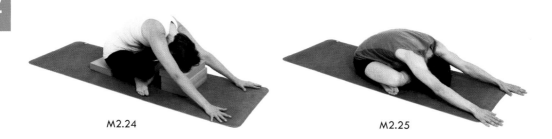

M2.24   M2.25

Savasana

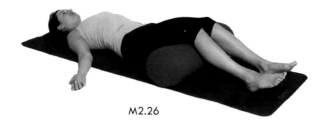

M2.26

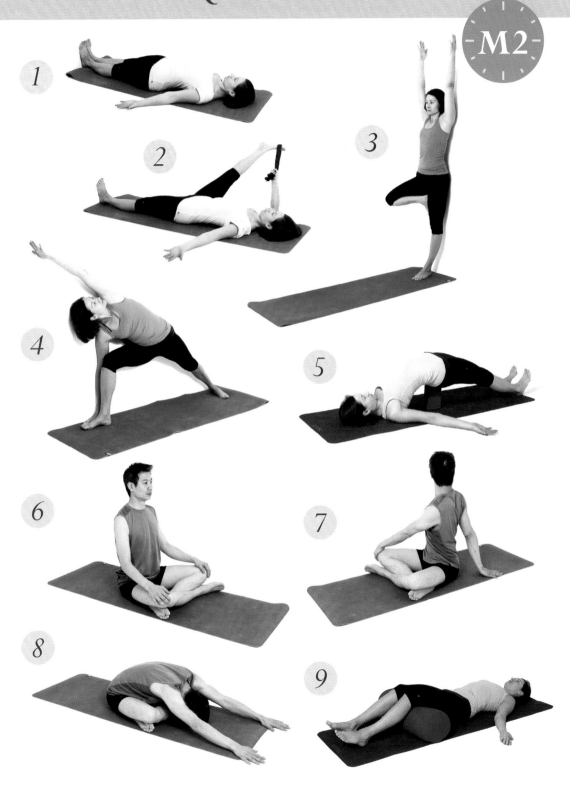

M2

M3 | MEDIUM PROGRAMME 3

*A sequence to strengthen the legs and arms, mobilise the spine
and hips, and tone the abdominal and back muscles*

YOU WILL NEED:
* A wall or flat support, or a chair or ledge

YOU MAY NEED:
* Blocks
* A chair or stool, roughly at knee height

Adho Mukha Svanasana

Downward facing dog

If you choose, you can do this once as you have been practising, with the hands on
a support, to remind yourself of how the legs have to work to take the weight out
of the hands, and to warm up the ankles, shoulders, wrists and hips. Then try it with
the hands on your mat.

* Kneel down. Spread the fingers well, and have the middle fingers pointing
  forward. Tuck the toes under and lift the hips high, then press the top of the
  thighs back to straighten the legs.

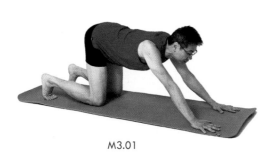

M3.01

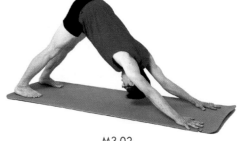

M3.02

- Extend the outer hips up and back, away towards the armpits, to create length on the sides of the body.
- Move the muscles of the shoulders away from the ears.
- Let the head and neck hang down.

Preparation for Virabhadrasana 1

Warrior 1

If you can't step the foot forward easily in this posture, you can help the knee forward with your hand, until the foot is between the hands.

If you find that the shoulders are hunched in this position, rather than the chest extending forward, have the hands on supports.

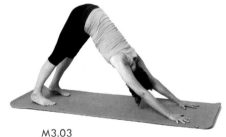

M3.03

- Be in Adho Mukha Svanasana. Look forward, and step your right foot centrally between your hands. Make sure that the ankle is under the knee. Keep your back leg straight, and stretch your heel away *(M3.05)*. Draw the left hip forward and the right hip back, so the hips are aligned. Move your tailbone deeply into the body. Reach your chest bone forward, and look forward *(M3.06)*.

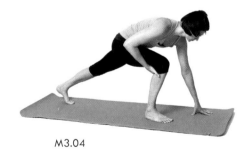

M3.04

- Step the front foot back to return to downward dog. Change sides.
- Repeat once more on each side.

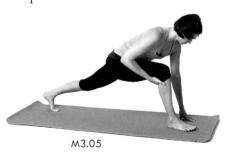

M3.05

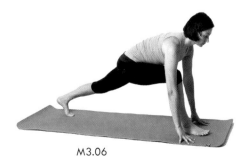

M3.06

M3

Uttanasana, going forward

Intense stretch pose

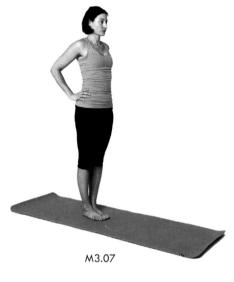

M3.07

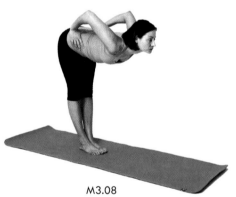

M3.08

If you find it hard to keep the spine extending and the legs straight in this posture, have the hands on a support. Have some blocks on your mat ready.

•   Stand in Tadasana. Lift the arch of the foot from its centre to feel the inner knees and inner thighs lift up. Move the tailbone in.

•   With the fingertips on the hips, extend the chest bone forward, hinging from the hips *(M3.08)*. Keep the kneecaps and thighs well lifted. Take the hands either to the floor *(M3.09)* or to the support *(M3.10)*. The spine should be extending, with the upper back slightly concave – if the back curves up to the ceiling, have the hands on a higher support.

•   Look forward, and lengthen the front body and the spine forward. To come up, place the fingertips on the hips, lift the thigh muscles and abdomen, and extend the chest bone forward and up to come back to a standing position.

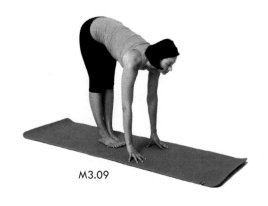

M3.09

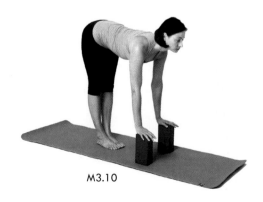

M3.10

Parivrtta Ardha Chandrasana, with support for the back foot

Revolving half-moon posture, or a standing balancing twist

If you needed support for your hands in Uttanasana, you will also need it for this posture. Have it ready towards the front (narrow) end of your mat.

Have a wall behind you so that you can place the foot up on it. You can use a chair or ledge instead if that's easier. At first, it might be tricky to get the right height and distance from the support, but find a position where you can keep both legs straight and extend the spine.

- Be in Uttanasana going forward, as in *M3.11*. Take your left toes back onto the mat behind you. Keep the hips level, and the thigh muscles well lifted.
- Lift the back heel up to place the sole of the left foot on the wall, with all the toes pointing down *(M3.12)*. (If you are using a chair or ledge, place the underside of the toes on it.)
- Have the foot in line with the hip – or if that's not possible, just as high as you can manage, keeping the leg straight.
- Keep the standing leg straight. Lift the arch of the foot from its centre, and feel that the inner knee and inner thigh lifts up. Extend the chest forward.
- From here, take your left hand across to where your right hand is, and take your right hand to your sacrum *(M3.13)*. Turn your abdomen to the right – towards the standing leg. Turn the waist, the diaphragm, and the chest fully to the right, then stretch the top hand to the

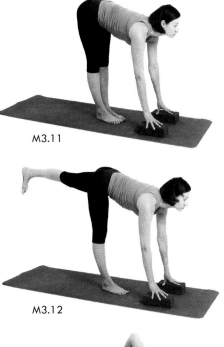

M3.11

M3.12

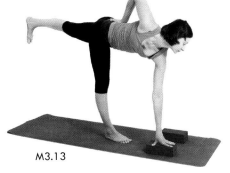

M3.13

M3

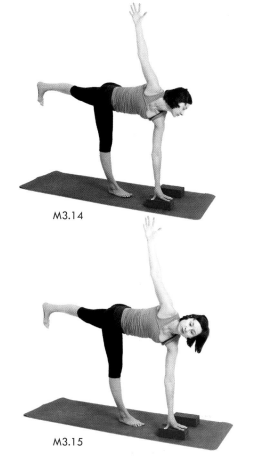

M3.14

ceiling *(M3.15)*. Reach the hands away from each other, and turn more. If you have your balance, look up *(M3.16)*.

• To come out of this posture look down, place the hands down, release the leg down, and change sides.

M3.15

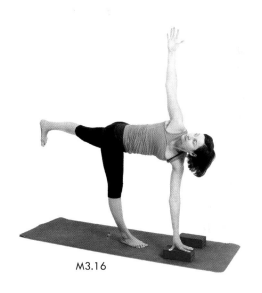

M3.16

Malasana

Garland posture, or squatting pose

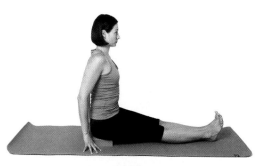

M3.17

If the heels do not reach the floor in this posture, place a firm support under the heels. Have a block or rolled blanket ready.

• Sit in Dandasana. Bend the legs one at a time, to come to a squatting position with the feet together and the soles of the feet on the floor *(M3.19)*. Stretch the arms out in front of you. Widen the knees, and extend the arms forward *(M3.20)*. At the

M3

same time, extend the outer thighs from the hip to the outer knee, and grip them towards each other.

- Take the hands to the floor, and lengthen the abdomen and sides of the body forward. Bend the left arm underneath the left shin, so that the hand reaches towards the heels, then do the same on the right side.

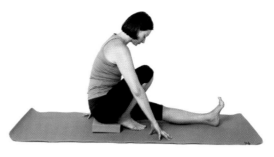

M3.18

- Reach the hands back, and clasp the heels *(M3.23)*. Release the head and neck down. Lift the shins up and hit them back so that there is a depth in the groins and an extension of the spine.

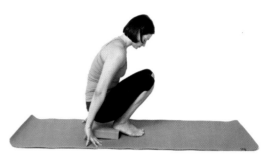

M3.19

- To come out of this posture, release your hands, look forward, extend your arms forward, and sit down. Extend the legs out in Dandasana.

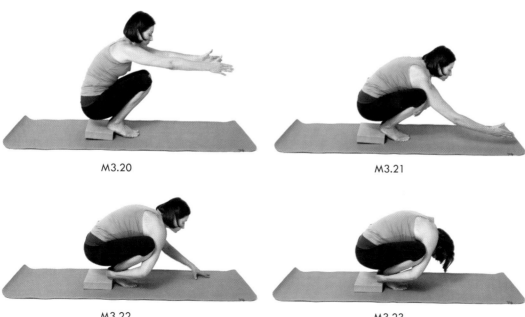

M3.20

M3.21

M3.22

M3.23

M3

BENEFITS:
Malasana
- Strengthens and tones the leg and abdominal muscles
- Improves circulation in the lower legs and feet
- Strengthens the ankles
- Stimulates the digestive system
- Lengthens and broadens the back body
- Improves flexibility in the hips and ankles
- Relieves anxiety and brings quietness to the mind

Kurmasana

Tortoise posture – a deep forward bending pose

If you are quite stiff in the back, hamstrings or hips, you might find that you need some support in this posture. It can be useful to sit up on a support if you find it difficult to lift your lower back in seated positions. If your hips or hamstrings are tight, you might find that having some support under the feet allows you to get deeper into this position. If the head doesn't easily come to the floor, have a support for the head, so that you can rest the head and neck down.

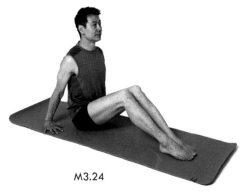

M3.24

Only go to the stage that is appropriate for you. If you feel that you can no longer go any deeper, then rest the head down and just stay in the position you have reached for a few minutes.

• Sit with the knees bent, and the feet on the floor, in front of the knees.

Stage 1

• Lengthen the abdomen and side trunk forward. Take your left arm underneath your left knee, and your right arm underneath your right knee *(M3.25)*.

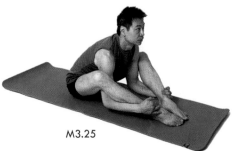

M3.25

Stage 2

- Extend the hands away, and reach the heels away, so that the legs are straighter and the chest is drawn forward *(M3.26)*.
- Rest the head down.

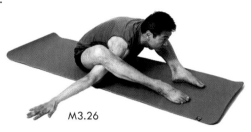

M3.26

Stage 3

- Walk the hands back towards your hips.

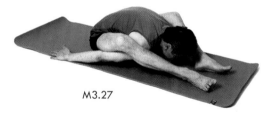

M3.27

Stage 4

- Bring the feet towards each other, then cross the ankles. Tuck your head in between your feet. Soften and broaden the back body *(M3.28)*.
- Clasp the hands behind the lower back *(M3.29)*.
- To come out of this, gently unclasp the hands and walk them forward. Undo the

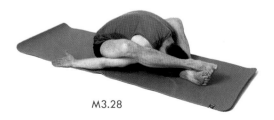

M3.28

feet and take them a little apart. Ease the body up off the floor and bring the hands in. Come back to Dandasana. Stretch the legs out straight in front of you.

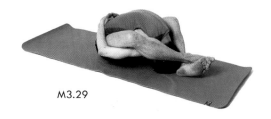

M3.29

Kurmasana, with support

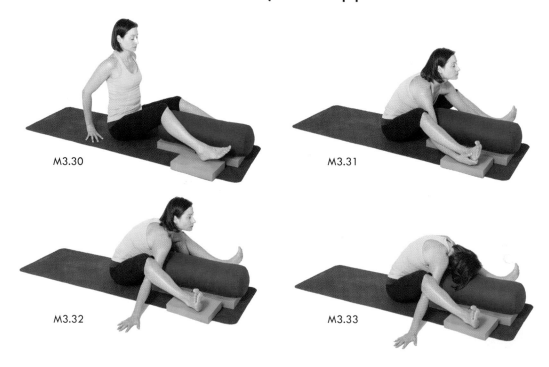

M3.30

M3.31

M3.32

M3.33

Savasana

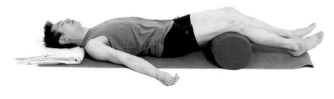

M3.34

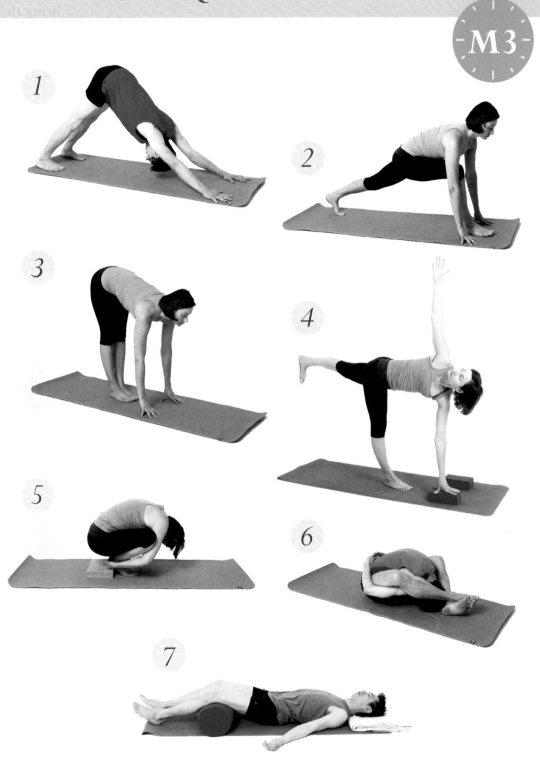

M3

1

2

3

4

5

6

7

M4 | MEDIUM PROGRAMME 4

*A sequence to increase flexibility in the spine,
tone the abdomen and back muscles,
stimulate the digestive system and open the chest*

YOU WILL NEED:
- A wall or vertical support
- A chair or stool
- A bolster or large cushion

YOU MAY NEED:
- A belt

Viparita Karani

*Inverted action pose,
or lying with the legs up the wall*

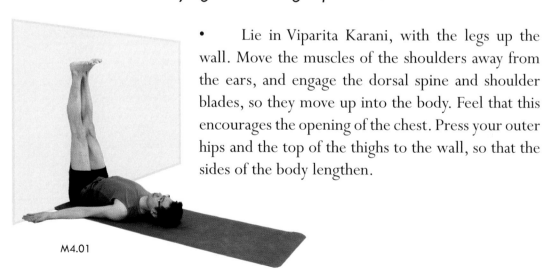

M4.01

- Lie in Viparita Karani, with the legs up the wall. Move the muscles of the shoulders away from the ears, and engage the dorsal spine and shoulder blades, so they move up into the body. Feel that this encourages the opening of the chest. Press your outer hips and the top of the thighs to the wall, so that the sides of the body lengthen.

Supta Tadasana

Supine mountain pose, practised with the feet to a wall

- Lie down, with the knees bent, and the soles of the feet close to a wall.
- Straighten the legs, and press the feet into the wall so that the body is pushed away from the wall. Feel that with this action the shoulder muscles are pulled away from the ears, and the flesh of the buttocks lengthens to the heels.
- With the feet together, reach the inner edges of the balls of the feet

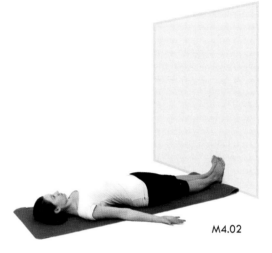

M4.02

into the wall. Feel that all four corners of the knees are facing the ceiling. If you lose the feeling of the feet pressing into the wall at any stage, bend the legs, move closer to the wall, and straighten the legs again, so that the feet stay active against the wall through the posture and the arm variations. The action of the feet helps to maintain the correct work in the legs and abdomen.

Arm Variations

Variation 1

- Stretch your fingers to the floor behind your head, with the palms facing each other, shoulder width apart.

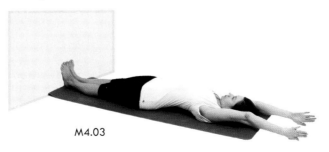

M4.03

M4

Variation 2

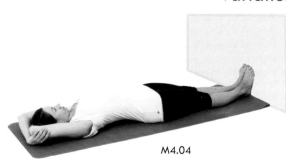

M4.04

• Clasp the elbows behind your head. Draw the corners of the elbows away from you, but keep the shoulders moving away from the ears. Engage the shoulder blades up towards the chest, and feel the elbows release down more. Move the tailbone to the heels, and feel that the abdomen releases down to the spine.

• Release, change the cross of the forearms, and repeat on the other side.

Variation 3

• With the fingers interlaced, take the hands towards the floor behind your head. Extend the thumb side of the hands away more. Draw the pubic bone to the navel, the navel to the chest bone, and the chest bone to the chin.

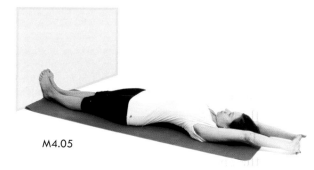

M4.05

• Release, change the interlacing of the fingers, so that the other thumb is on top, and repeat.

Jathara Parivartanasana, resting

Revolved abdomen pose, or supine twist

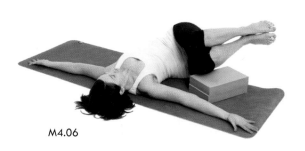

M4.06

For a gentler version of this posture, or if the knees don't easily come to the floor, have some support under the knees (M4.06).

• Lie down with the knees bent, and the feet flat on the floor. Have

M4

the knees and feet together. Move the shoulders away from the ears, and reach the tailbone towards the heels, so the abdomen releases down to the spine *(M4.07)*.

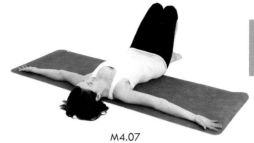

M4.07

- Take the arms wide, in line with the shoulders. Stretch the fingers away from each other. Bring the knees in to the chest, and squeeze the knees together. Reach the fingers of the left hand away more strongly, and take the knees to the right elbow. Release them down towards the floor.

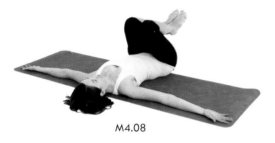

M4.08

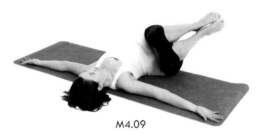

M4.09

- Keep the knees releasing towards the floor, and reach the left hand away more. Turn the abdomen to the ceiling and reach the chest to the left hand.

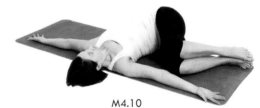

M4.10

- To come back to the starting position, draw the abdomen back to the spine and bring the knees up to the chest, then practise to the other side. Repeat once again on each side.

Jathara Parivartanasana, active

Revolved abdomen pose, or supine twist

Here, the posture is practised as a fluid movement, with the knees staying off the floor. This means the work becomes more abdominal. When the knees are down and the posture is a resting one (as in the previous variation), there is more depth to the spinal action.

- Lie down in Supta Tadasana. Bend the knees, keeping the knees and feet together.

M4

Stretch the arms out to the sides.

- Bring the knees towards the chest, keeping them together, then bring the knees to the right elbow, or as close as they will go – but don't let them touch the floor. At the same time, reach the left fingers away more. Draw the abdomen to the spine and bring the knees back to centre, then repeat to the other side. Make this a fluid action – don't go too quickly or too slowly. Keep the face quiet and looking at the ceiling, and the shoulders away from the ears. Repeat five times to each side. To finish, lie with the knees bent and the soles of the feet on the floor.

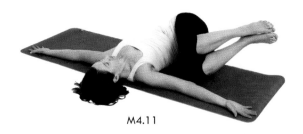

M4.11

Preparation for Parivrtta Trikonasana

Revolving triangle posture, or a standing twist with the legs straight

- Be in Adho Mukha Svanasana (downward dog) with your hands on a chair *(M4.12)*.

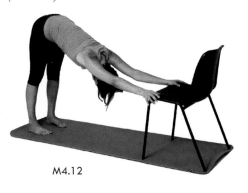

M4.12

- Look forward, and step the right foot forward. Straighten the legs, and broaden the back of the left thigh to reach the left hip forward, so the hips are level. Extend the chest bone forward. Move your left hand to the centre of your support, so it is in line with your chest bone, then take your right hand to your sacrum *(M4.13)*. Pin your back heel down, and turn your abdomen to the right. Open the right shoulder to the ceiling, and engage the left shoulder blade into the body to turn the chest to the ceiling. Stretch the right hand up to turn the chest and abdomen more *(M4.14)*.

M4

- To come out of this posture, look forward, replace the hands on the chair, and step back to your downward dog. Change sides.

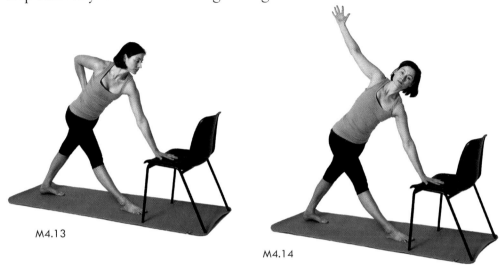

M4.13

M4.14

Parivrtta Trikonasana

Revolving triangle posture, or a standing twist with the legs straight

You may need some support for your hand — if you do, or if you're not certain, have a block ready towards the front (narrow) edge of your mat.

- Stand in Tadasana at the back edge of your mat *(M4.15)*.
- Have your fingertips on your hips. Turn your left toes out a little, and step your right foot forward. Broaden the back thigh of the back leg, to draw the hip forward. Take the front hip back, so the hips are level. Lift the sides of the body *(M4.16)*.
- Keep the hips level and the thigh muscles well lifted. Extend the chest bone and the front body forward, then take your left hand to the floor to the outside of your right shin *(M4.17)*. If you can't take the hand to the

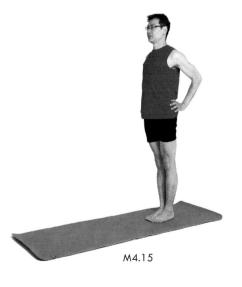

M4.15

M4

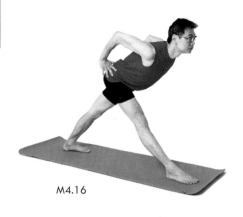

M4.16

floor, take it onto a block.

• Extend the pubic bone to the navel, the navel to the chest bone, and the chest bone to the chin.

• Turn your abdomen and chest to the right, and then up towards the ceiling.

• Pin your back heel down, and turn your abdomen more. Open the right shoulder to the ceiling, and engage the left shoulder blade into the body to turn the chest to the ceiling. Reach the right hand up *(M4.18)*.

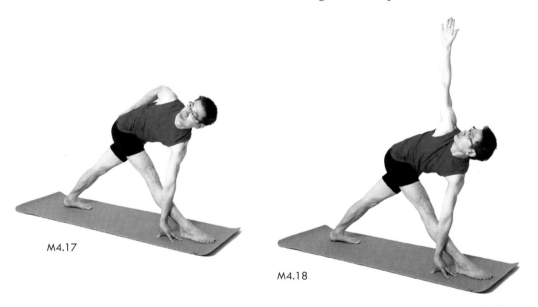

M4.17

M4.18

• You can keep the gaze down at the front big toe until you have found your balance. When you feel you have stability in the posture, and the turn of the spine is coming well, then you can gradually turn the head, until you are facing up to the top hand.

• To come up, look down, and bring your top hand down to your hip. Take your left hand off the floor or the block and bring it to your left hip. Extend the front body forward, keep the legs firm, and lift back to standing. Step your back foot forward, then come back to Tadasana at the back of your mat to do the other side.

Ustrasana

Camel pose,
or kneeling backward bending posture

If the ankles are stiff and you find kneeling in this way uncomfortable, or if there is a gap under the shins, have some padding under the ankles, shins and knees.

Variations

Variation 1 – with a chair

- Kneel up, with the knees and feet hip width apart. Have a chair behind you, and sit with your feet slightly underneath the front of the seat. Feel that the weight is on the centre line of both shins and the top of the ankles *(M4.19)*.

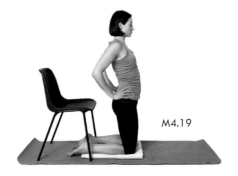

M4.19

- Lift the front thigh muscles and the thigh bones up. Move the tailbone firmly into the body, and lift the pubic bone up, so that the abdomen and chest also lift.
- Pull the shoulder muscles away from the ears, and reach your hands back until you catch the sides of your chair. Move the shoulders blades and dorsal spine into the body, then lift and curve your chest up and back. Feel that the sides of the chest are lifted and open *(M4.20)*.

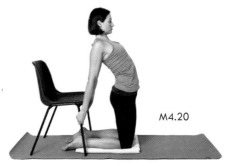

M4.20

- Keep the lower part of the posture very active to support the work in the upper body: press the shins and ankles down, and lift the thigh muscles and pubic bone up *(M4.21)*.

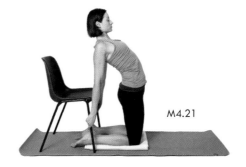

M4.21

- Lift your chest bone up more, then finally

M4

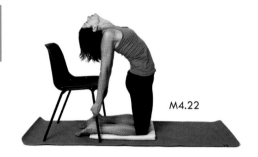

M4.22

release the head back *(M4.22)*. The throat should stay soft: if it feels like it is over exposed, or the chest drops, stay looking forward.

- To come up, keep the chest lifting to the ceiling, and press your shins down to lift back to a vertical position – bring the head up last. Sit down on the heels for a moment to rest.

- If you felt that this variation with the chair was strong enough, then repeat it or move on to the next posture – Supta Tadasana. If you felt that it was comfortable, try the next variation.

Variation 2 – with a bolster or cushion

- Kneel up as in variation 1, but instead of the chair, place a bolster or large cushion over the backs of your ankles. Lift the front thigh muscles and the thigh bones up. Move the tailbone firmly into the body, and lift the pubic bone up. Place your hands onto the back of your buttock crease and pull the shoulder muscles away from the ears. Move the shoulders blades and dorsal spine into the body, then lift and curve your chest up and back. Pull the shoulder muscles away from the ears more. Feel that the sides of the chest are lifted and open *(M4.24)*.

- Reach your hands back to the bolster *(M4.25)*, then lift your chest bone up more, and finally release the head back *(M4.26)*.

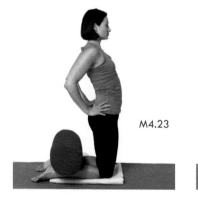

M4.23

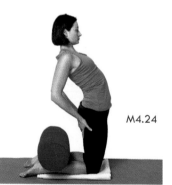

M4.24

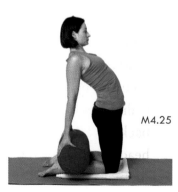

M4.25

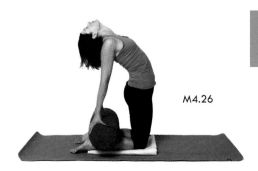

M4

- To come up, keep the chest lifting to the ceiling, and press your shins down to lift back to a vertical position – bring the head up last. Sit down on the heels for a moment to rest.

M4.26

- If you felt that this variation with the bolster was strong enough, you can either repeat it or move on to the next posture – Supta Tadasana. If you felt that it was comfortable, try the next variation.

Variation 3 – final posture

- Kneel up, with the knees and feet hip width apart. Lift the inner thigh muscles up. Lift the pubic bone up, so that the abdomen and chest also lift. Place your hands onto the backs of your buttock crease and draw the shoulder muscles away from the ears. Move the shoulders blades and dorsal spine into the body, then lift and curve your chest up and back. Press your shins and ankles down firmly and lift the inner thighs and the pubic bone up more *(M4.27)*.
- Reach your hands back to your heels one at a time *(M4.28)*, then lift your chest bone up more, and finally release the head back *(M4.30)*.
- To come up, keep the chest lifting to the ceiling, and press your shins down to lift back to a vertical position – bring the head up last. Sit down on the heels for a moment to rest.

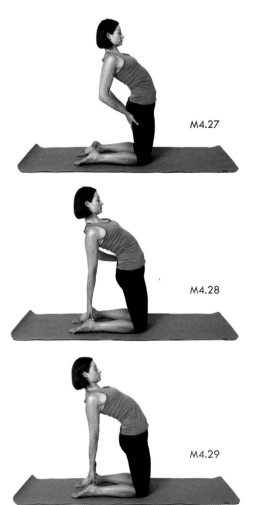

M4.27

M4.28

M4.29

M4

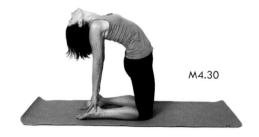

M4.30

FOCUS ON: The downward
action of the shins and ankles,
to create lift in the posture

Even though it might feel tempting, do not curl up into a ball or do a forward bend
after a strong back bend like this. Firstly, you should allow your body to feel the
back bend fully, rather than immediately erase it. Secondly, the spine needs to be
brought back to a neutral position before you bend forward — which is why the
next postures are spinal extensions and twists.

Supta Tadasana

Supine mountain posture

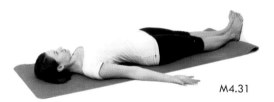

M4.31

- Lie down in Supta Tadasana for several moments, to allow the spine to lengthen.
  You can stretch the arms over the head to extend the spine more strongly if you
  choose.

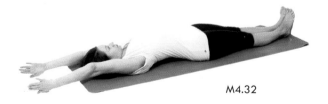

M4.32

Jathara Parivartanasana, resting

Revolved abdomen pose, or supine twist

This can be done with support for the knees, to make the action less strong, or without.

- From Supta Tadasana, bend the knees and place the knees and feet together. Grip the knees in. Feel that this draws the outer thighs and outer hips together. Stretch the arms out wide *(M4.33)*.

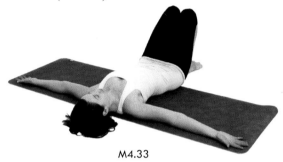

M4.33

- Bring the knees towards the chest, keeping them together, then bring the knees to the right elbow. Reach the left fingers away. Rest the knees down on the floor or on the support close to the elbow. The knees should be as close to the line of the shoulders as possible, so the stomach muscles are not strained. Turn the abdomen to the ceiling, away from the bent legs. Turn the chest to the left hand. Move the skin and flesh on the back body to the right. Keep the face looking at the ceiling – the neck turns easily, so concentrate on turning the rest of the spine fully.
- Draw the abdomen back to the spine to bring the knees back to centre. Repeat to the other side. To finish, lie with the knees bent and the soles of the feet on the floor.

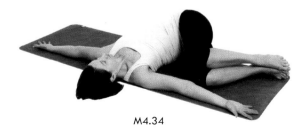

M4.34

Viparita Karani, resting

M4

- Before you go up into Viparita Karani, place a bolster or long cushion near to the wall (about a fist's distance away from it), and have a folded towel or blanket to hand for your head.
- To come into the posture, lie on your side with your lower hip on the very edge of the bolster *(M4.36)*, then roll up as normal. When you are in the right position, the back of the sacrum will be supported on the bolster *(M4.37)*, allowing the rest of the spine to lengthen without effort. Place the folded blanket under your head and neck.

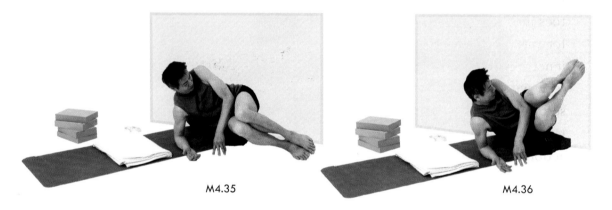

M4.35

M4.36

- Release the muscles of the shoulders away from the ears, and engage the dorsal spine and shoulder blades, so they move up into the body. Reach the balls of the feet firmly to the ceiling. The bones of the thighs move down into the hip

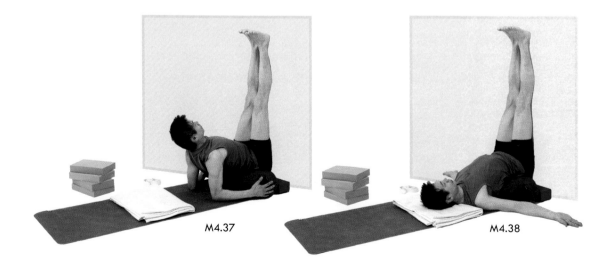

M4.37

M4.38

sockets. Move your outer hips and the very top part of your thigh to the wall, so that the sides of the body lengthen.

- Place yourself well for the posture, as you have practised previously, and feel that having placed yourself correctly you can relax without losing the essence of the posture.

Adho Mukha Virasana

Child's pose

- Kneel with the knees a little apart and the big toes just touching. Lengthen the chest bone forward, so the abdomen extends along the inner thighs. Rest the hands back by the feet, with the palms facing up. Broaden and soften the back body. If you wish, you can take support under the head to make the action gentler.

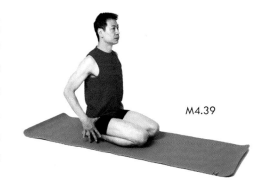

M4.39

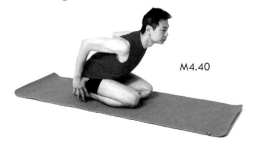

M4.40

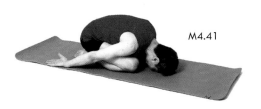

M4.41

Savasana

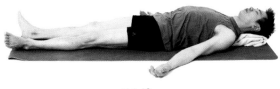

M4.42

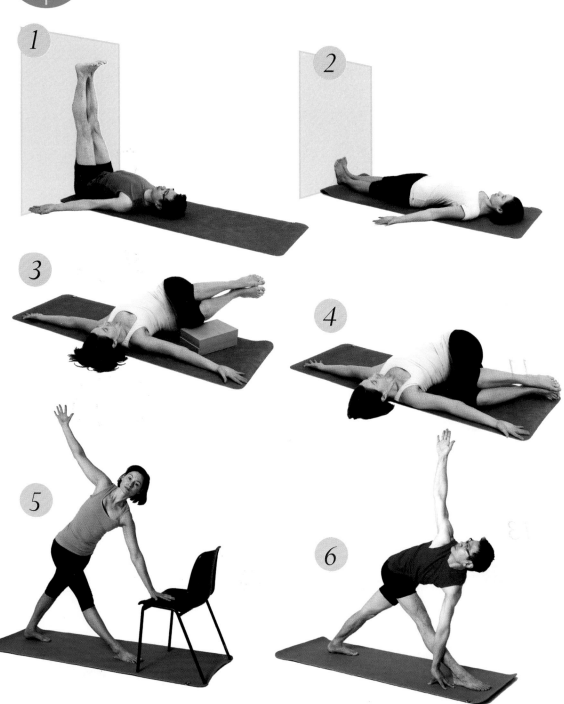

M4

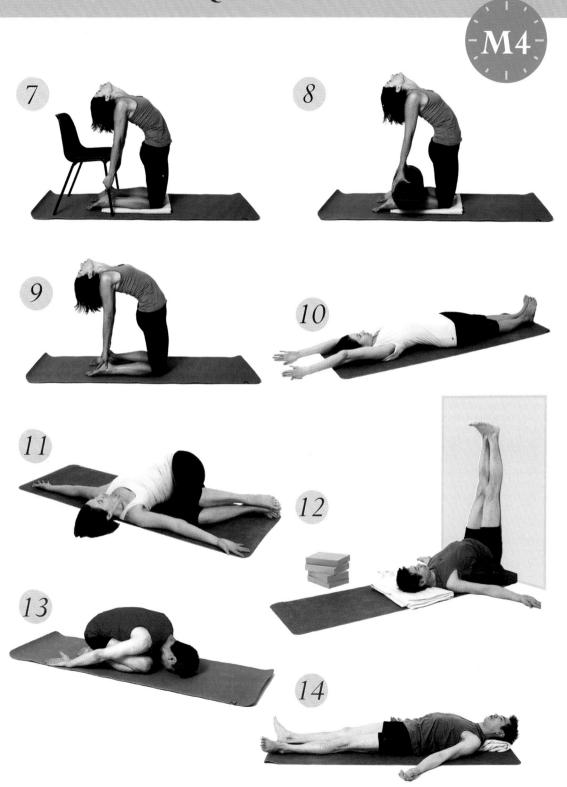

M5 | MEDIUM PROGRAMME 5

A sequence to strengthen and tone the arms and legs, improve balance, tone the abdomen and increase mobility in the hips, shoulders and spine

YOU WILL NEED:
- A chair or other support that is roughly hip height
- A wall or vertical support
- A long cushion or bolster, or a folded blanket

YOU MAY NEED:
- A belt

Tadasana with Urdhva Baddhanguliyasana and Gomukhasana

Tadasana with arm variations (backward extension, upward bound fingers pose and cow face pose)

- Stand in Tadasana.

Arm Variations

Variation 1

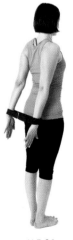

M5.01

- If you are using a belt, put it around your wrists, behind your back. Stretch your fingers, and reach the hands back and down *(M5.01)*. Keep the tailbone moving into the body, and draw the lower abdominal muscles up and then back to the spine. Feel that the abdominal muscles are pliant, and broad. Maintain this feeling of lift and breadth, so that the posture becomes lighter.

Variation 2 – Urdhva Baddhanguliyasana

- Take the hands into Urdhva Baddhanguliyasana. Keep the shoulders away from the ears, the tailbone moving into the body, and the lower abdomen lifting up and drawing back.
- Release, change the cross of the fingers, and repeat *(M5.02)*.

Variation 3 – Gomukhasana

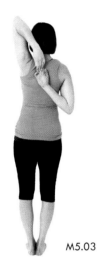

- Take the arms into Gomukhasana, with the right arm down. Keep the chest bone lifted, and the corner of the right shoulder back, so that the body stays upright, with even length on both sides of the torso *(M5.03)*. Release and change sides.

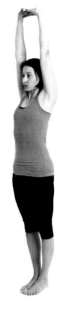

M5.02

M5.03

FOCUS ON: **The action of the tailbone and lower abdomen**

Adho Mukha Svanasana

Downward facing dog

If you choose, you can do this once as you have been practising in the short sequences, with the hands raised.

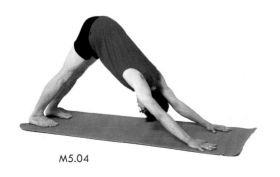

M5.04

- Be in Adho Mukha Savnasana.
- Roll your back armpit to your front armpit. Lift the muscles of your front thighs up and press them back, away from your hands. Engage the abdominal muscles back towards the spine, but maintain the feeling of breadth and

M5

pliancy in the abdomen.
• Let the head and neck hang down.

Preparation for Virabhadrasana 1

Warrior 1

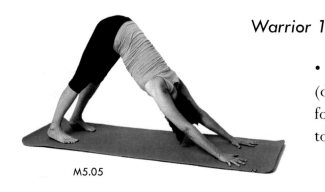

M5.05

• Be in Adho Mukha Svanasana (downward dog). If you need support for the hands, have a few blocks ready towards the front of your mat.

Variations

Variation 1

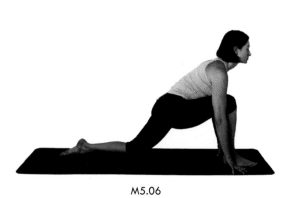

M5.06

• Look forward, and step your right foot centrally between your hands. Have the ankle under the knee – do not let the knee overshoot the foot. Bend your back knee and place it on the floor, and turn your toes backwards. Draw the left hip forward and the right hip back, so the hips are aligned. Move your tailbone deeply into the body. Draw the shoulder muscles away from the ears, reach your chest bone forward and look forward.

• Tuck your back toes under and step the front foot back to return to downward dog. Repeat on the other side.

Variation 2

M5

- Be in downward dog. Look forward, and step your right foot centrally between your hands. Have the ankle under the knee. Keep your back leg straight, and stretch your heel away. Draw the left hip forward and the right hip back, so the hips are aligned. Move your tailbone deeply into the body. Draw the shoulder muscles away from the ears, reach your chest bone forward, and look forward.
- Step the front foot back to return to downward dog. Repeat on the other side.

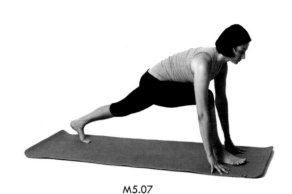

M5.07

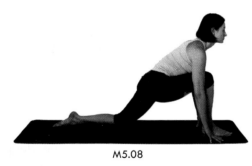

M5.08

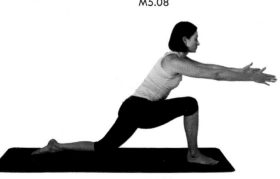

M5.09

Variation 3

- Come to the forward extension in Variation 1. From here, draw the lower abdomen back to the spine, extend the arms forward then up, to bring the spine to vertical. Reach your hands to the ceiling. Have the palms facing and the hands shoulder width apart, and keep the shoulders away from the ears. Stamp your back shin into the floor, move the tailbone in and lift the pubic bone and the chest bone. Lift the abdomen up, and draw it back to the spine.

M5

- To come out of this, keep the abdomen engaged. Reach the arms and chest bone forward, place the hands back down, step back to downward dog, then repeat on the other side.

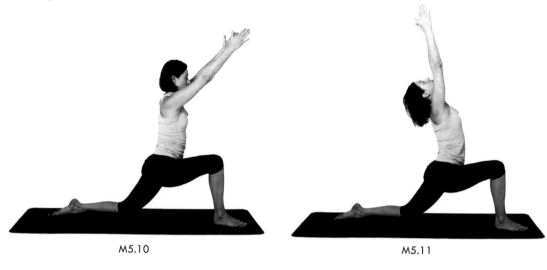

M5.10

M5.11

Variation 4

- From variation 2, draw the lower abdomen back to the spine, then extend the arms forward then up, to bring the spine to vertical. Reach your hands to the ceiling. Have the palms facing and the hands shoulder width apart. Keeping the hips level, press your back heel away, move the tailbone in and lift the pubic bone and the chest bone. Keep the abdomen moving back to hold the spine, and lift it up more.
- To come out of this, reach the arms and chest bone forward, place the hands back down, step back to downward dog, then repeat on the other side.

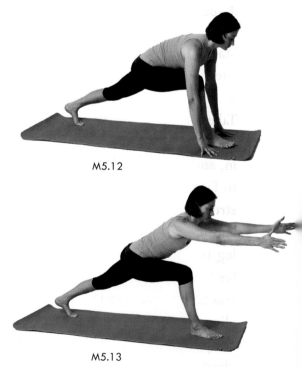

M5.12

M5.13

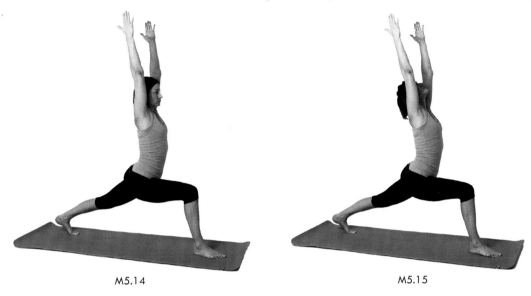

M5.14   M5.15

Virabhadrasana 1

Warrior 1

If you have a back or knee problem, just step the legs apart — don't jump.

- Stand in Tadasana in the middle of your mat. Take the fingertips to the chest and step or jump the legs wide apart, stretching the arms out at shoulder height *(M5.18)*. Take your arms up into Urdhva Hastasana. Turn your left foot well in, and your right leg fully out. Turn to face the right leg. Keep the hands stretching up, and lift the chest bone and the abdomen up. Bend the right leg to a right angle *(M5.21)*. Pin the back heel down, and keep the left hip reaching forward to that the hips stay aligned. Move the tailbone in, lift the pubic bone up, and finally lift the chest more and look up.

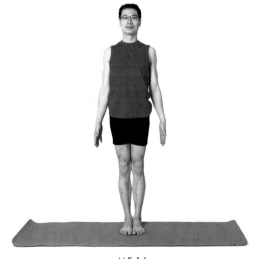

M5.16

M5

- To come up, look forward. Pull the hands to the ceiling and straighten the front leg. Turn your feet to face forward, then jump or step the legs together to come back to Tadasana. Repeat to the other side.

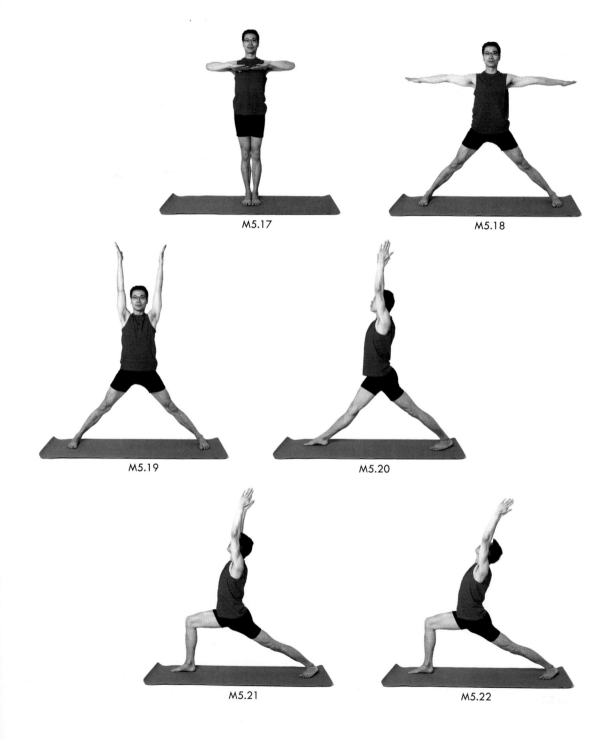

M5.17

M5.18

M5.19

M5.20

M5.21

M5.22

Virabhadrasana 3

Warrior 3

If you choose, you can do the preparatory version of this posture first (as shown in S6), with the hands against a wall or ledge, to remind yourself of the alignment. Then try the full version.

If you have a back or knee problem, just step the legs apart – don't jump.

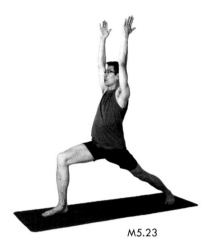

M5.23

- From Virabhadrasana 1, as above, look forward and reach the arms forward. Step the back toes in a little, then straighten the front leg and left the back leg to hip height – or, if that's not possible, just as high as it will go. Keep the fingers reaching forward, and draw the chest bone forward. Extend the ball of the back foot away. Lift the abdomen to your spine, and keep it broad.

- To come out of this, bend the front leg, step the back foot back and come back to Virabhadrasana 1. Pull the hands to the ceiling to straighten the front leg, turn to face forward, then jump or step the feet together.

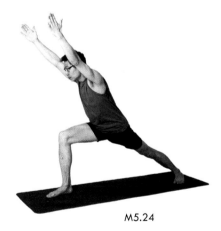

M5.24

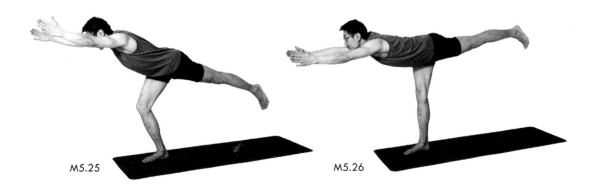

M5.25   M5.26

Marichyasana 3 Variation

M5

Marichyasana is named after a sage
Standing twist, with the foot raised

- Start in Tadasana *(M5.27)*. Lift the muscles of the thighs and move them back, onto the bones of the thighs. Take the weight into the heels. Move the tailbone into the body; feel the abdomen and spine lift.

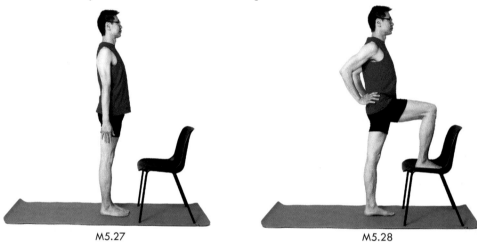

M5.27   M5.28

- Bend the right leg, raise the foot and take it up onto your support. Have the heel underneath the knee, and the knee in line with or higher than the hip *(M5.28)*.
- Lengthen the outer hip down, so that the hips are level. Grip the hips together.
- Turn towards the bent leg. Take the back of the left hand onto the outside of the

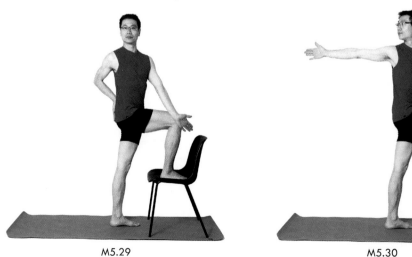

M5.29   M5.30

right leg. Press the hand against the leg and the leg against the arm to turn the abdomen. Stretch the right arm away *(M5.30)*.

- Draw your left thigh muscle up and back onto the bone of the thigh, so that your hips stay level.Lift the abdomen and chest. Turn to the right. Start the twist from the lower abdomen, then turn the waist, the diaphragm and the chest. Let the head follow the turn of the spine.
- To release, look forward then turn forward. Change sides.

Supta Swastikasana, with the feet supported

Supine cross-legged posture

This is a very restful posture for the legs and back, so should feel particularly nice after the strong standing sequence.

- Lie down, as if for Savasana, but with the backs of the knees over a bolster or folded blanket. Move the shoulder muscles away from the ears so the chest is opened, and move the flesh of the buttocks and the tailbone away from the waist so the spine is lengthened. From here, cross the legs so the feet rest on the cushion, and the knees release down. Rest the backs of the hands on the floor, or place the hands on the abdomen.
- After a few moments, release and change the cross of the legs.

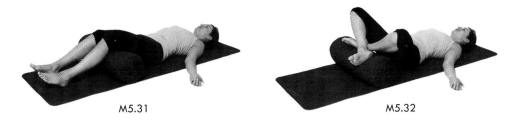

M5.31   M5.32

Savasana

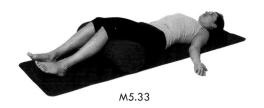

M5.33

A Quick Reminder

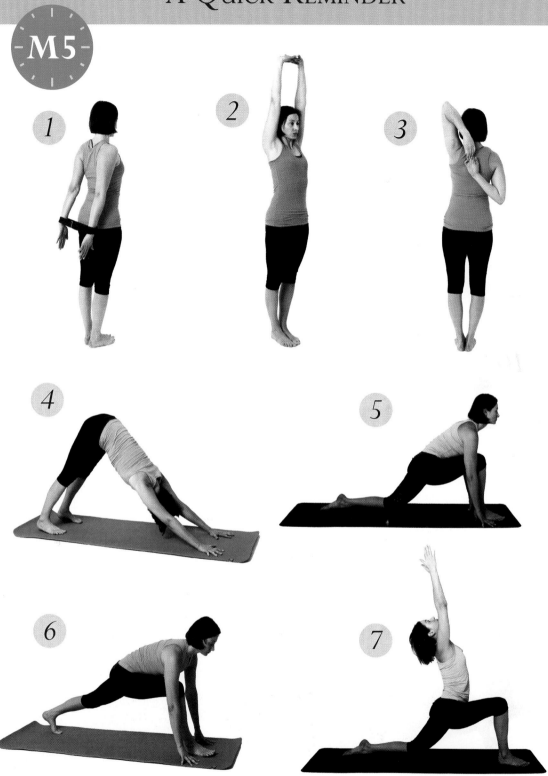

M5

1

2

3

4

5

6

7

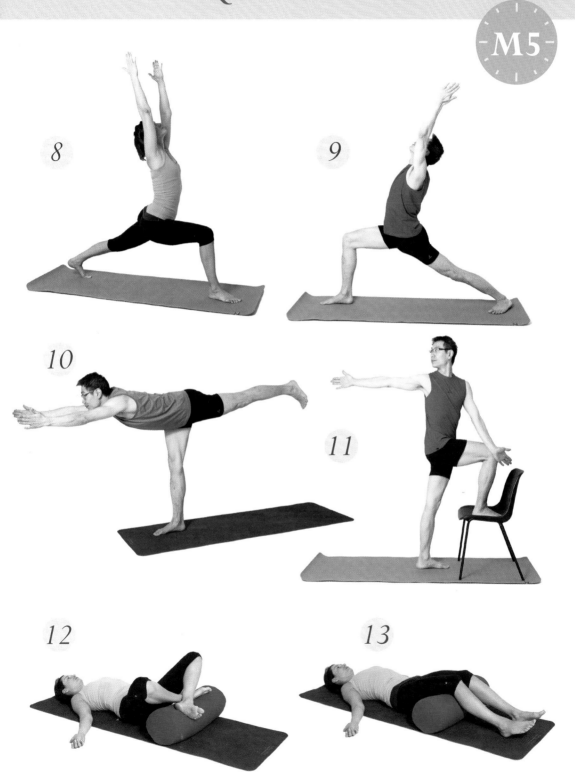

M6	MEDIUM PROGRAMME 6

A sequence to improve flexibility in the hips, ankles, shoulders and wrists, improve circulation in the legs and tone and strengthen the abdominal, leg and back muscles

YOU MAY NEED:
- A belt
- A wall or vertical support
- Blocks or cushions, or a folded towel or blanket

Tadasana with Urdhva Baddhanguliyasana, Gomukhasana and Paschima Namaskarasana

Mountain pose with upward bound fingers, cow and reverse prayer positions

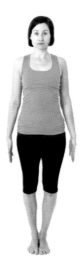

- Stand in Tadasana.
- Pull the central arches of the feet and the inner knees up. Pull the inner thighs to the groin *(M6.01)*.

Arm Variations

Urdhva Baddhanguliyasana

- Take the hands into Urdhva Baddhanguliyasana. Keep the abdomen moving back, and lifting up.
- Release, then change the interlacing of the fingers, so that the other thumb is on top, and repeat *(M6.02)*.

M6.01

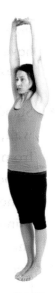

M6.02

Gomukhasana

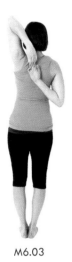

• Take the hands into Gomukhasana, with the left arm lifted. Lift the front armpit on the side of the lower arm, and draw the corner of the shoulder back. Release, and change sides *(M6.03)*.

Paschima Namaskarasana

• Take the hands into Paschima Namaskarasana. Open the corners of your shoulders back. Pull the muscles of your upper arms down to the corners of the elbows, and lift your front armpits up *(M6.04)*.

M6.03

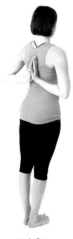

M6.04

Utkatasana

Difficult or awkward pose,
or standing with the legs bent and the arms raised

Practise this against a wall to begin with. When you have the alignment and the lift of the body, try it freestanding.

• Stand in Tadasana, with your back against the wall, and your feet about thirty centimetres away from it. Grip the outer thighs together. Move the tailbone in, and draw the abdomen back to the spine, and up. Hold the diaphragm back to the spine, and broaden it. Feel that there is strength and lift on the core of the body.

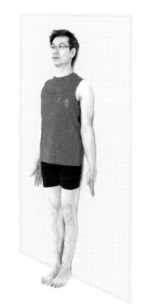

M6.05

• Bend deeply at the ankles and hips and slide the body down the wall, until the knees are in line with

M6

the hips and the thighs are parallel to the floor. Stretch the arms up, keeping the hands shoulder width apart, with the palms facing. Lift the chest bone and the abdomen strongly *(M6.07)*.

- To come out of this posture, pull the hands to the ceiling and push the feet into the floor to bring yourself back to standing.

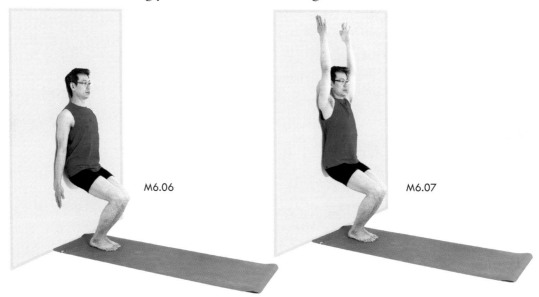

M6.06   M6.07

Utkatasana

Freestanding

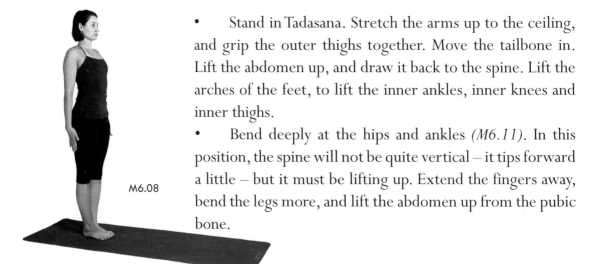

M6.08

- Stand in Tadasana. Stretch the arms up to the ceiling, and grip the outer thighs together. Move the tailbone in. Lift the abdomen up, and draw it back to the spine. Lift the arches of the feet, to lift the inner ankles, inner knees and inner thighs.
- Bend deeply at the hips and ankles *(M6.11)*. In this position, the spine will not be quite vertical – it tips forward a little – but it must be lifting up. Extend the fingers away, bend the legs more, and lift the abdomen up from the pubic bone.

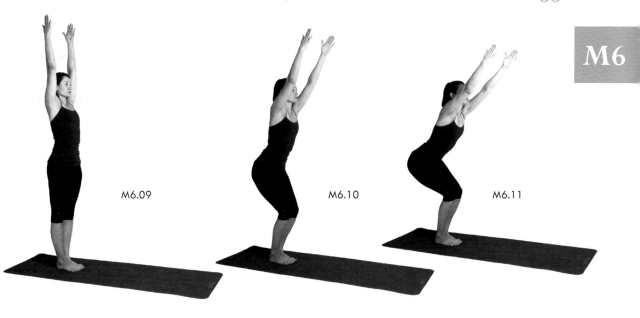

M6.09 M6.10 M6.11

M6

Garudasana

Eagle pose, or standing balancing with the arms and legs bound

Practise this against a wall to begin with. When you have the alignment and the lift of the body, try it freestanding.

- Stand in Tadasana, with your back against a wall, and your feet a short distance away from the wall. Lift the arches of the feet from the centre, keeping the inner big toe joint moving down. Lift the thigh muscles and inner knees.
- Bend at the ankles and hips, as if you were coming into an easy version of Utkatasana, then lift the right knee up. Cross the top of the thigh as high up over the left as it will go, and wrap the right foot around the back of the left calf. If it won't go that far, just take the toes as far around as possible.

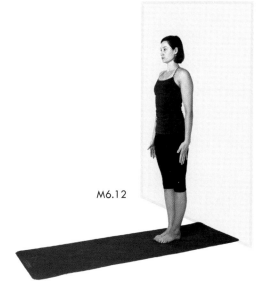

M6.12

M6

- Stretch the arms out at shoulder height. Because the right leg is on top, the left arm is on top, for balance. Swing and cross the left upper arm over the right, then bring the backs of the hands together, with the thumbs pointing towards your face. Scissor the hands so that the palms touch. Reach the shoulder muscles away from the ears, and broaden your collar bones. Lift the elbows and the chest bone up, and move the hands away from the face.

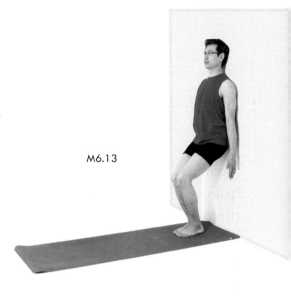

M6.13

- Draw the right hip back, so the sacrum is aligned on the wall both horizontally and vertically. Lift the inner arch of the foot and the inner knee of the standing leg, so that the standing leg doesn't collapse inward. Keep the tailbone in, and lift the abdomen up.
- Release the arms then the legs to come back to Tadasana. Change sides.

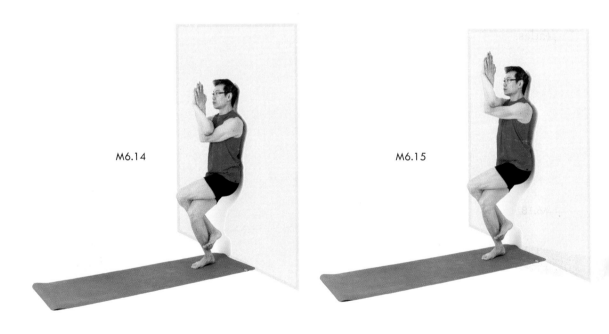

M6.14

M6.15

Garudasana

Freestanding

- Stand in Tadasana. Stretch the arms out at shoulder height. Swing and cross the left upper arm over the right *(M6.16)*, then bring the backs of the hands together, with the thumbs pointing towards your face. Scissor the hands so that the palms touch *(M6.18)*. Reach the shoulder muscles away from the ears, and broaden your collar bones. Lift the elbows and the chest bone up, and move the hands away from the face.

- From here, bend deeply at the ankles and hips *(M6.19)*, then lift the right leg up and over the left *(M6.20)*. Cross the top of the thigh as high up over the left as it will go, and wrap the right foot around the back of the left calf *(M6.21)*.

- Lift the inner ankle, inner knee and inner thigh of the standing leg, and draw the right hip back to keep the hips and sacrum level. Stretch the arms up more, and lift the chest bone.

- Release the arms first, then the legs, to come back to Tadasana. Change sides.

M6.16

M6.17

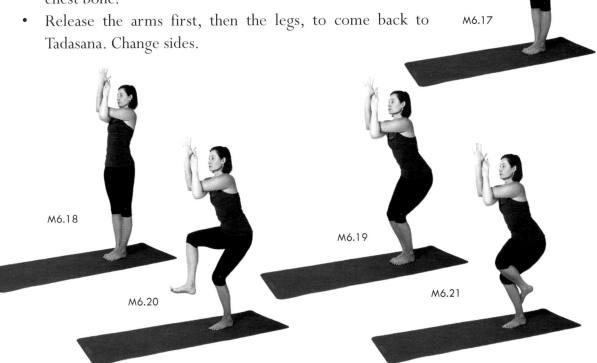

M6.18

M6.19

M6.20

M6.21

Urdhva Prasarita Padasana

M6

Upward extended feet pose, or lying supine with the legs raised

This posture works the abdominal muscles strongly, but it also requires flexibility in the hips and hamstrings. If you find that you can't lift the legs in this way, or there is a lot of shaking in the legs or body, keep your hands by your hips, with the palms turned down. Don't hold the posture for too long.

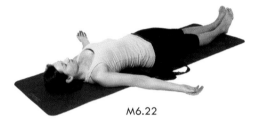

M6.22

- Lie in Supta Tadasana. Move the shoulders away from the ears, and lengthen the tailbone to the heels, so the abdomen moves down. Stretch the arms over the head *(M6.23)*.
- Bend the knees into the chest *(M6.24)*, then stretch the legs to the ceiling. Extend the fingers away, and keep the balls of the feet reaching up. Hold the abdomen down to the spine, and keep it broad *(M6.25)*.
- Bend the knees, and release the feet to the floor.
- Repeat twice.

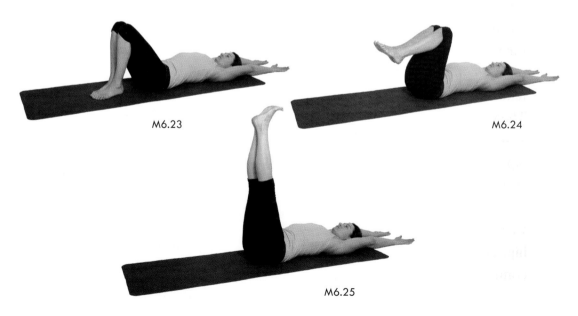

M6.23

M6.24

M6.25

Ardha Matsyendrasana

Matsyendrasana is named after a sage
Half-seated twist

If it isn't possible to sit on the heels, have support under the buttocks. There should be no pain in the knees. If you have knee problems, make sure you support the knees, as shown in S3.

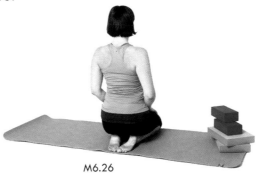

M6.26

Variations

Variation 1

- Kneel as you would for Virasana, but with the knees and feet together *(M6.26)*.
- Sitting up a little, displace your right foot forward. The left buttock bone should be on the heel, but if this isn't comfortable take support under the buttock bone. The right buttock bone is floating, so take a firm support underneath it so that the hips are level. Draw the right hip joint down and suck the hips in towards each other.

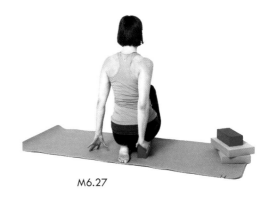

M6.27

- Cross your right leg over the left, bringing the foot towards its opposite hip. The right foot can point forward, or turn out a little, whichever is most comfortable. Grip the legs together.

M6

• Press the right hand into the floor behind you, and lift the spine up. Lift the left arm up, turn the abdomen to the right, and cross the left arm onto the outside of the right leg, keeping the arm straight.

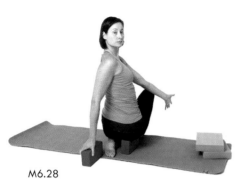

M6.28

• Press the front arm into the leg to turn your abdomen fully to the right. Resist the leg back against the arm, to keep the knee upright. Turn the abdomen to the right. Turn the circumference of the ribs and chest to the right. Keep the corners of the shoulders back, and the chest bone well lifted. Let the head follow the turn of the spine.

• Look forward, then release. Change sides.

Variation 2

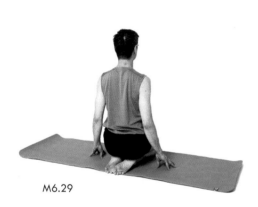

M6.29

• Sitting up a little, displace your right foot forward, and turn your left foot in, so that the little toe side of the foot is on the mat, pointing to the right. Sit your right buttock bone on the ball of the left foot, and the left buttock bone on the inside of the heel. If you feel unsteady or uncomfortable, put some support or some padding on top of the foot. Draw the right hip joint down and suck both hips in.

• Cross your right leg over the left, bringing the foot towards its opposite hip. Grip the legs together.

• Place the right hand into the floor behind you, and lift the spine up. Lift the left arm up, turn the abdomen to the right, and cross the left arm onto the outside of the right leg.

• Bend the arm, and lift the front armpits up. Press the arm against the leg to turn the chest and abdomen. Resist the leg against the arm to keep the knee upright. Turn the abdomen fully

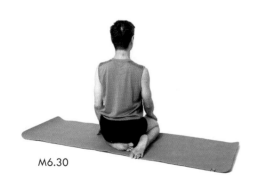

M6.30

to the right. Turn the circumference of the ribs and chest. Keep the corners of the shoulders back, and the front body well lifted.

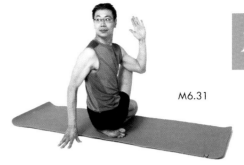

M6

- Look forward, then release. Change sides.

M6.31

Marichyasana 3

Marichyasana is named after a sage
A seated twist

If you find it difficult to sit with the legs straight and the back upright in Dandasana, sit up on a support for this posture.

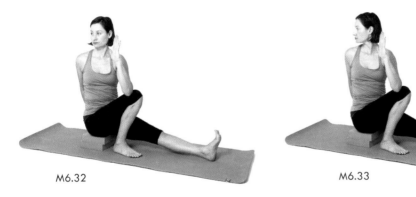

M6.32   M6.33

- Sit in Dandasana *(M6.34)*. Bend the right leg, so the heel touches the buttock. Have the heel in line with its own buttock bone *(M6.35)*.
- Take the right hand back, and press it down to lift the spine up. Reach the left arm up, turn the abdomen to the right, and cross the arm over the right leg. Bend the arm, and press the bent arm against the leg. Lift

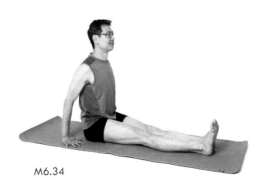

M6.34

the front armpits up, and turn to the right. Resist the leg against the arm to keep the knee upright and to deepen the turn of the abdomen. Turn the chest. Keep the front body well lifted, and the collar bones broadening. Allow the head to follow the turn of the spine *(M6.36)*.

- Look forward, then release. Change sides.

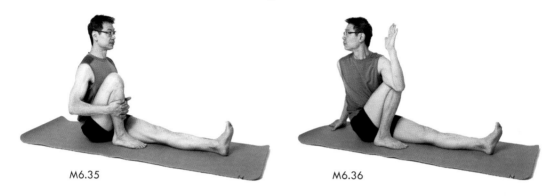

M6.35   M6.36

Adho Mukha Virasana

Virasana is named after a sage
Kneeling with the head down, or child's pose

If it isn't possible to sit on the heels, have support under the buttocks. If your forehead doesn't reach the floor, or you find you're straining to bring it down, take some support for the forehead.

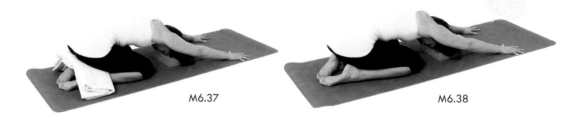

M6.37   M6.38

- Sit on your heels.
- Take your fingers under the underside of each knee, where it meets the shin, and draw it forward. Then place the hands under the feet and draw the toes back and the top of the feet back *(M6.39)*. Do this several times, lengthening

M6

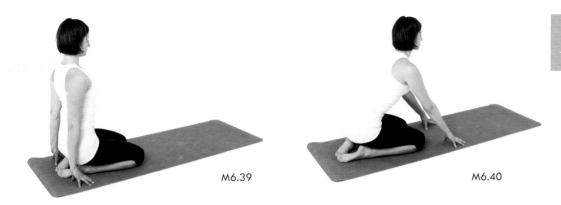

M6.39   M6.40

the shin bones forward and the feet back, and opening the ankle joint to the floor.

- Place your hands on the floor in front of your knees *(M6.40)*, and use your hands on the floor to press your buttocks down to the heels. The buttock bones and tailbone move down and point down *(M6.41)*.
- Then come into Adho Mukha Virasana.
- Have the hands wider than your shoulders, and spread your fingers. Rotate the upper arm muscles from the inside to the outside, but at the same time pin the inner wrist side of your hand down. Let the head and neck rest *(M6.42)*.

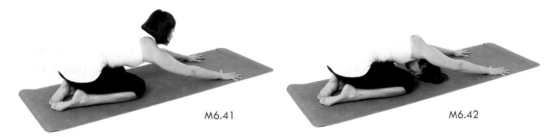

M6.41   M6.42

Savasana

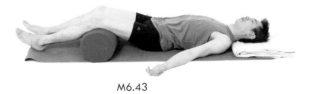

M6.43

A Quick Reminder

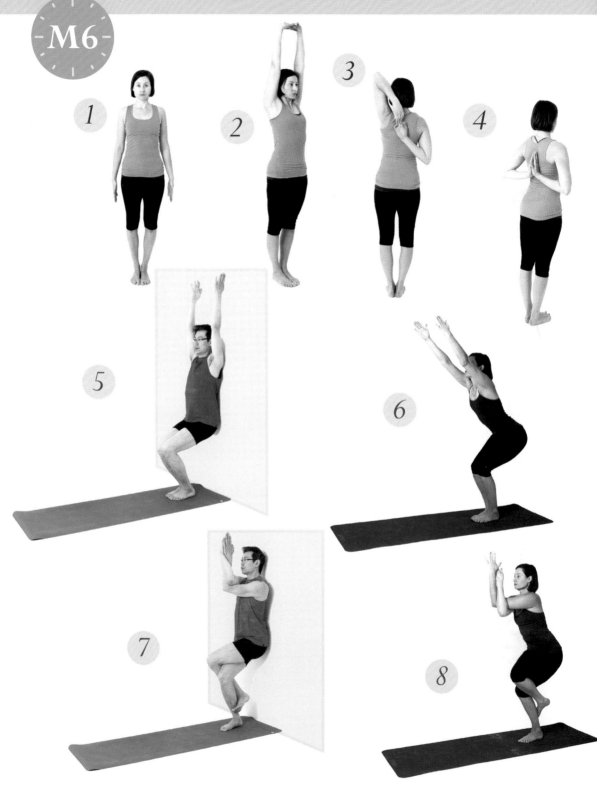

M6

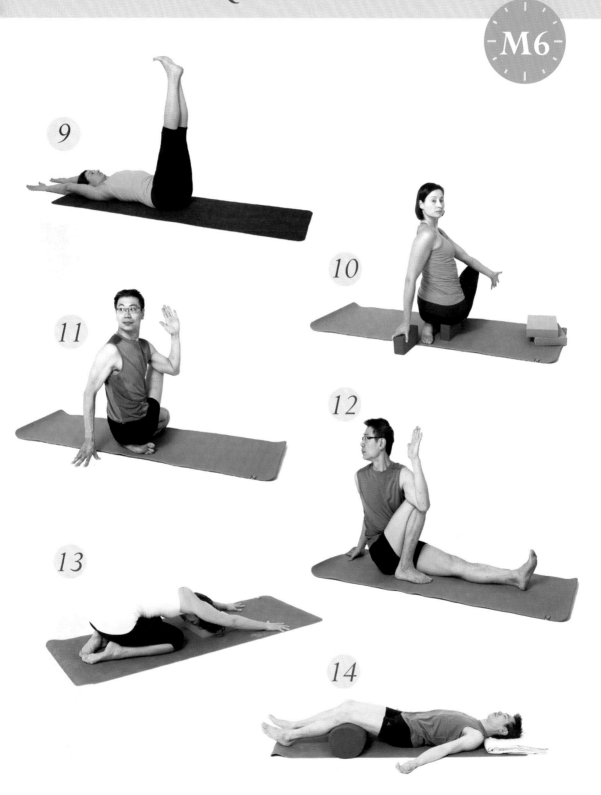

9

10

11

12

13

14

M7 | MEDIUM PROGRAMME 7

*A sequence to strengthen and mobilise the wrists
and ankles, create openness in the shoulders
and chest, and lengthen the spine and abdomen*

Adho Mukha Virasana
and Parsva Adho Mukha Virasana

*Virasana is named after a sage. Kneeling with the head down
Sometimes known as child's pose. Parsva means to the side*

If it isn't possible to sit on the heels, have support under the buttocks. If the head doesn't come to the floor, take some support under the forehead, so the neck can relax.

• Be in Adho Mukha Virasana, with the arms outstretched. Pin the buttock bones down.

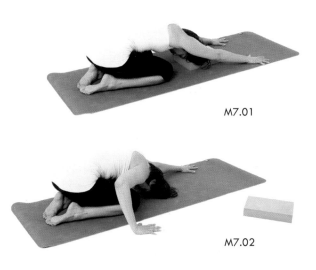

M7.01

M7.02

• From here, reach your left hand across to where your right hand is, and move your right hand to the outside of your right knee – with the fingers pointing forward (*M7.03*). Extend the left hand away and press it down, and use that action to pin the left buttock bone down more, so that the left side of the body extends. Press the right hand into the floor, lift your abdomen and turn it so that it rests on the right thigh. Place the forehead in front of the right knee (*M7.05*). Keep the left buttock bone pinned down, and the abdomen turning onto the thigh.

- Move the hands back to their original positions and bring yourself back to centre. Change sides.

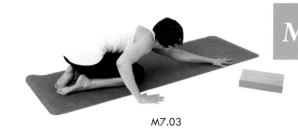

M7

M7.03

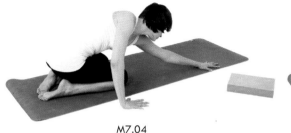

M7.04

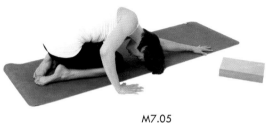

M7.05

Uttanasana

Intense stretch pose

You may need some support under the hands *(as in M7.06 and M7.07)* – if you do, or if you're not certain, have a couple of blocks ready.

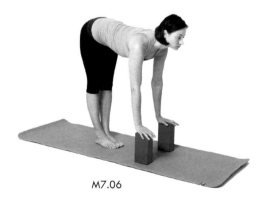

M7.06

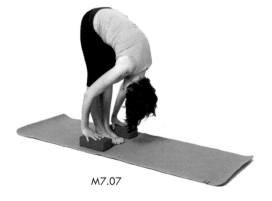

M7.07

- Come into Uttanasana from Tadasana. Place your hands by the outside edges of your feet *(M7.11)*. Grip the outer ankles in, and lift the inner ankles, inner knees and inner thighs strongly up. Reach the chest bone and the front armpits to the floor, and lift the back thighs.
- Bend your elbows back, and draw the sides of the body down. Keep the

M7

shoulders away from the ears. Lift and separate the buttock bones. Let the head and the neck hang down.

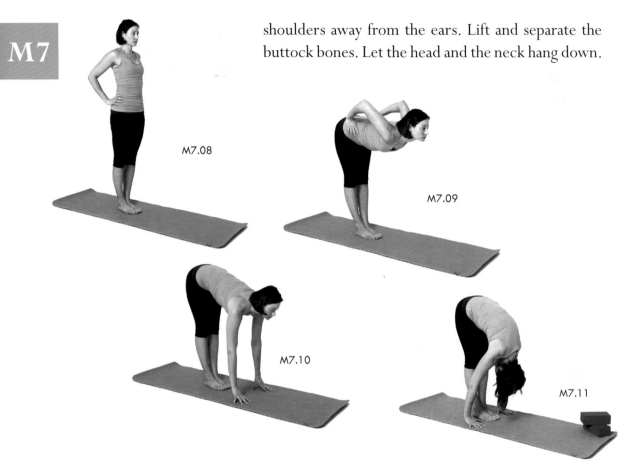

M7.08

M7.09

M7.10

M7.11

Uttanasana Variation

Intense stretch pose, with the back to a wall

If you are stiff in the hamstrings or back, you'll need to start with the feet a little further away from the wall – try this once or twice until you get the right distance.

Don't twist as you come into this posture or come out of it – bend the knees and press the hands against the wall to come into and out of the posture.

- Stand facing a wall. Bend the knees, place the hands on the wall, and walk the hands down

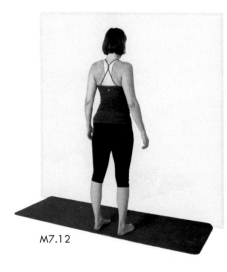

M7.12

the wall. Tuck your chin in and place the back of the shoulders against the wall. Walk the hands down, then place the hands on the floor and straighten the legs. Lean into the wall, and slide yourself further down, lifting the buttock bones up as you do so. Keep the heels pinning down *(M7.14)*.

- If you go down quite far, you can rest the backs of the hands on the floor. Open the backs of the knees, lift the back thighs, and keep the front thigh muscles lifting strongly.

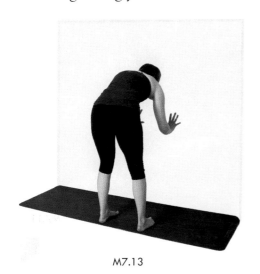

M7.13

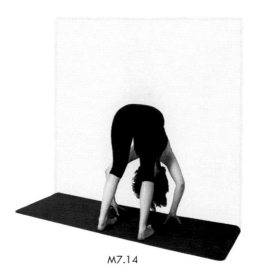

M7.14

- To come up, place your hands on the floor and take the weight into the hands. Bend the knees, and walk your hands up the wall to push yourself up. Bend the knees more, bring your head up, and come back to standing.

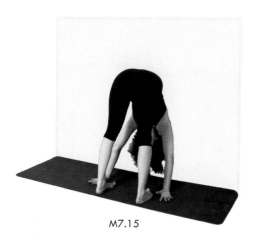

M7.15

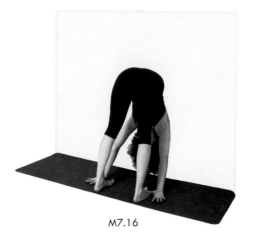

M7.16

M7

Utthita Hasta Eka Padasana

Extended hand to one foot posture
— sometimes known as standing split

Practise this first with the back toes to a wall or ledge, then try it freestanding. If you need support under the hands in Uttanasana, have it ready.

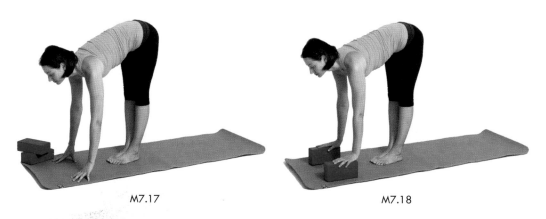

M7.17   M7.18

- Be in Uttanasana extending forward *(M7.17)*.
- Grip the hips together. Lift the left heel towards the ceiling, as high as you can comfortably take it *(M7.20)*. Place the back toes on a wall or support. Keep the hips level, and the back toes pointing down — if they turn out, it's a sign that the hips have come out of alignment. Extend the chest forward, then bend the elbows wide to reach the chest to the floor, and closer to the leg. Walk the hands back to the sides of the foot.

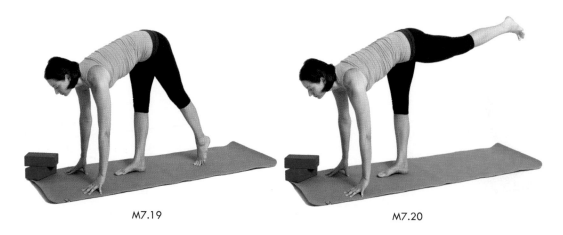

M7.19   M7.20

Variations

Variation 1

- Take the right hand to the right ankle. Use the hand against the ankle to draw the chest closer to the standing leg, and lift the back heel higher.

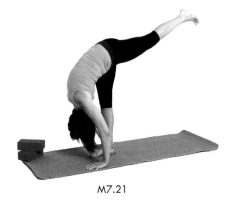

M7.21

Variation 2

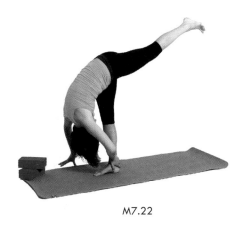

M7.22

- Take the left hand to the right ankle. Feel that this allows you to grip the hips in more, extend the spine further and lift the leg higher.
- Release, bring the feet together, and the hands back to the floor. Change sides.
- To come up, take the fingertips to the hips, grip the hips in and lift the abdomen up. Extend the chest forward and up to come back to Tadasana.

Adho Mukha Svanasana

Downward facing dog

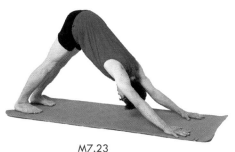

M7.23

- Be in Adho Mukha Svanasana.
- Lift the muscles of your front thighs up and press them back, away from your hands. Extend the inner thighs and the outer calves back.
- Rotate the muscles of the upper arms

from the inside to the outside, but keep the skin on the forearms rotating the other way – from the outside in. Grip the upper arms towards each other. Keep the base of all the fingers pressing into the floor, and move the shoulder blades in.

Chaturanga Dandasana

Four-limbed staff pose – a spine extending, balancing posture

Variations

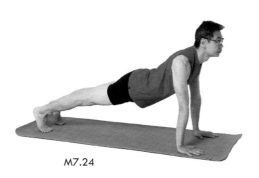

M7.24

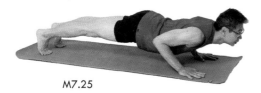

M7.25

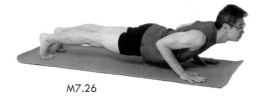

M7.26

Variation 1

• Be in downward dog, as in *M7.23*.
• Look forward. Move your weight forward, until your shoulders are above your wrists. This is known as plank position. Lengthen the back of your tailbone to your heels, and move your inner thighs and front thighs up. Press the heels back *(M7.24)*. Draw the abdominal muscles up, and make them broad.
• From here, bend your elbows back to your heels to come into Chaturanga Dandasana, hovering off the floor. Keep the thighs and abdomen engaged upwards, and the back of the tailbone extending to the heels. Pull the elbows back and extend the front armpits forward.
• Slowly release down to the floor, and rest the forehead down.

Variation 2

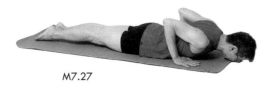

M7.27

• Lie prone, with the feet hip bone width apart with the toes tucked under, the forehead on the floor, and the hands by the lower ribs, with the fingers pointing forward. Press the heels back, and lift the thighs up off the floor. Engage the abdominal muscles towards the spine *(M7.28)*.

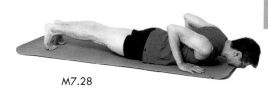

M7.28

- Draw the backs of the upper arms towards the elbows, and the corners of the elbows back to the heels.
- Look forward. Press the hands down, extend the chest bone forward, and the heels back, and lift the whole body off

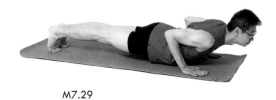

M7.29

the floor, so that just the hands and feet are in contact with the floor. Feel that the body is in one horizontal plane.

- Slowly release back to the floor, and rest the forehead down.

Bhekasana

Frog pose – a prone chest-opening position

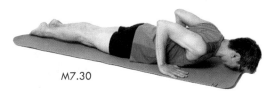

M7.30

- Lie prone, with the forehead on the floor. Place your hands next to your lower ribs, with the fingers pointing forward. Turn your toes back.
- Engage the tailbone down to the floor,

lengthen the abdomen and chest forward, and move the shoulder muscles away from the ears.

Stage 1

- Bend the right leg, and reach the right hand back to catch the foot. Place the hand so that the fingers reach to the ankle, and the heel of the hand presses into the toes. Open the right shoulder back, and draw

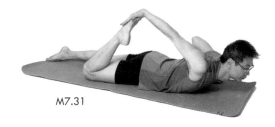

M7.31

M7

the foot down towards its own buttock, and then to the floor at the side of the hip. Lengthen the front armpit forward on both sides of the body, and keep the tailbone moving down. From here, look forward.

- Release, and change sides.

Stage 2

- From Stage 1, turn the fingers that are holding the foot out the side, and then to face forward, catching the toes with the heel of the hand. Feel that the arch of

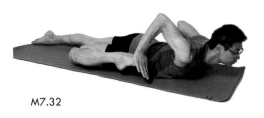

M7.32

the foot is activated. Press the other hand into the floor, lengthen the front armpits forward on both sides of the body, and keep the tailbone moving down. Look forward and extend the chest forward.

- Release, and change sides.

Stage 3

- Bend both legs, and catch the feet. Turn the fingers to point forward, as in variation 2, if that's possible. Look forward. Draw the backs of the upper arms towards the elbows.

- Press the feet down, lengthen the outer thighs away from the hips, and draw the inner thighs to the groins.

- Release down.

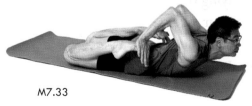

M7.33

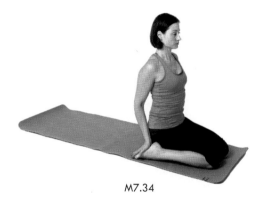

M7.34

Virasana

Kneeling position

- Sit in Virasana. Draw the diaphragm back, and lift the chest bone up. Feel that the back of the head is in line with the back of the sacrum.

Supta Virasana

Supine kneeling posture, with or without support

If it isn't possible to sit in Virasana with the buttocks on the floor or on a small support, continue to practise Virasana sitting upright rather than going back into the supine version. You may need to work with support under the back body in this posture. Have a bolster or some blocks and blankets ready behind you on your mat, as shown in M7.35.

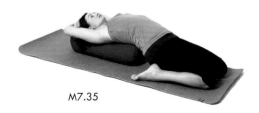

M7.35

- Sit in Virasana. Take the hands behind the hips, grip the hips in and lengthen the tailbone towards the backs of the knees to come back into Supta Virasana. Draw the frontal hip bones to your armpits. Reach the arms to the floor behind your head. If you're lying on a support, clasp your elbows behind your head; if you're lying flat, extend the arms out.
- Pin the shins down to lengthen the spine more. Draw the inner thighs to the inner groins, and extend the front body fully.
- To come up, take the hands to the feet. Press the elbows into the floor and lift up to kneeling. Stretch the legs out in front of you in Dandasana.

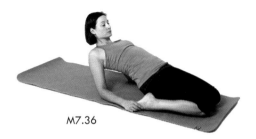

M7.36

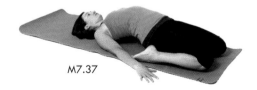

M7.37

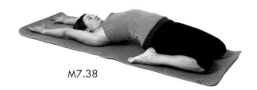

M7.38

Savasana

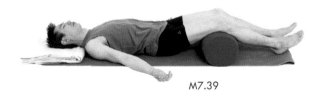

M7.39

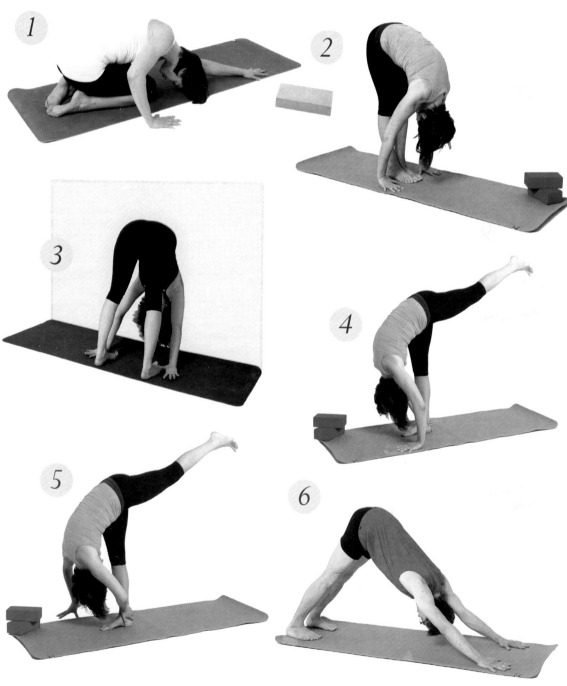

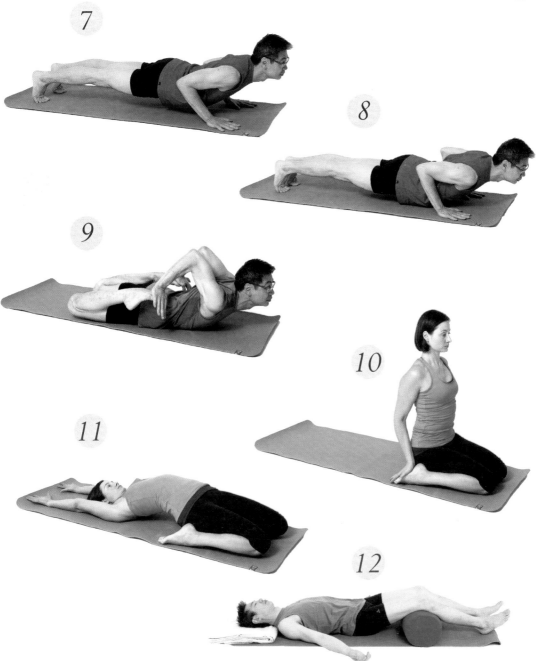

7

8

9

10

11

12

Long Programmes
35 - 45 minutes

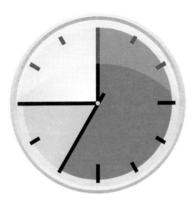

L1 | LONG PROGRAMME 1

A sequence to increase flexibility in the spine, open the chest and shoulders, tone the abdomen and back muscles, stimulate the digestive system and revitalise the body and mind

YOU WILL NEED:
- A wall, or ledge at roughly hip height

YOU MAY NEED:
- A belt
- Cushions, blocks or folded towels or blankets

Tadasana with Urdhva Baddhanguliyasana and Gomukhasana

Mountain pose, with upward bound fingers and cow face pose

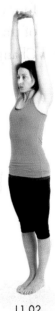

- Stand in Tadasana.
- Stretch your fingers back and down. Move the back ribs in, and lift the chest bone up. At the same time, draw your side ribs back. Extend all the toes. Lift the arches of the feet and the inner legs up. Grip the outer hips in *(L1.01)*.

Arm Variations

Urdhva Baddhanguliyasana

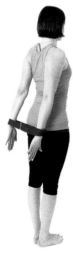

- Take the hands into Urdhva Baddhanguliyasana. Move the tailbone in. Engage the back ribs and the shoulder blades into the body, but draw the abdomen back to the spine *(L1.02)*. Release, change the cross of the fingers, and repeat.

L1.01

L1.02

Gomukhasana

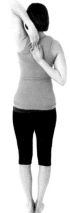

L1

- Take your arms into Gomukhasana, with the left elbow up. Draw the corner of the right shoulder back, and lift the right front armpit up. Move the shoulder blades into the body, but keep the abdomen drawing back to the spine. Release and change sides *(L1.03)*.

L1.03

Preparation for Virabhadrasana 3, with hands raised on a support

Warrior 3

- Start in Ardha Uttanasana, with the feet together. Grip the outer hips in. Keep the shoulder blades moving to the floor, and the abdomen lifting up, to hold the spine.
- Without disturbing your posture, take your left toes back.
- Keep your toes pointing down to the floor, and lift your left thigh up until the foot comes in line with the hip. Reach into the ball of the foot. Keep the thigh of the standing leg lifted and the outer hip reaching away from its own armpit.
- Change sides.

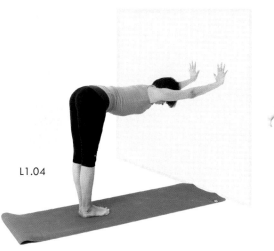

L1.04

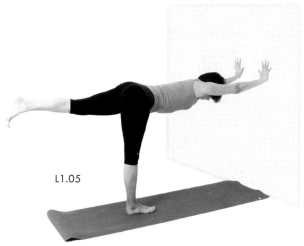

L1.05

Adho Mukha Svanasana

Downward facing dog

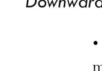

- Be in Adho Mukha Svanasana. Lift the muscles of your front thighs up and press them back, away from your hands. Draw the lower abdomen in. Grip the hips in, and extend the outer hips up and back.

L1.06

Virabhadrasana 1 and 3, from Adho Mukha Svanasana

Warrior 1 and 3, from downward facing dog

Warrior 1

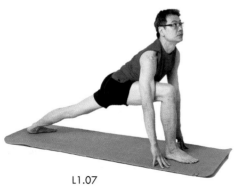

- From Adho Mukha Svanasana, as above, look forward, and step the right foot between the hands. Turn the back heel in towards the centre of the mat, and press it into the floor – but keep reaching the back

L1.07

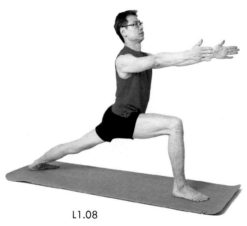

L1.08

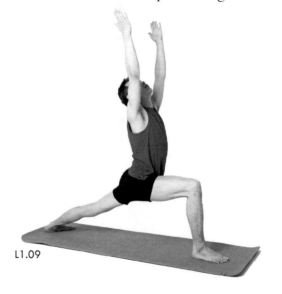

L1.09

hip forward, so that both hips are in one line. Hold the tailbone in, grip the hips in, and reach the arms forward, then up to the ceiling. Draw the lower abdomen in, and lift the abdomen and the chest up. Look up.

Warrior 3

- From Virabhadrasana 1, look forward. Extend the arms and chest bone forward. Step the back toes in a little, then straighten the front leg and lift the back leg to hip height. Press the ball of the back foot back, reach the fingers away, and hold the abdomen up towards the spine.
- To come out of this, bend the front leg, step the back foot back and come back to Virabhadrasana 1. Take the hands to the floor, and step back to downward dog.
- Change sides.

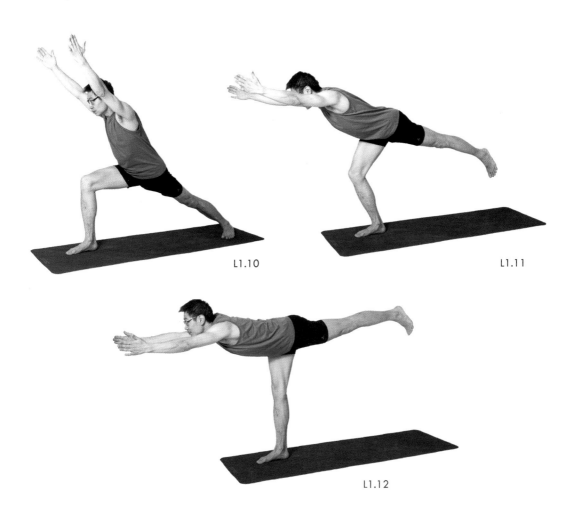

L1.10

L1.11

L1.12

L1

Salabhasana

Locust pose, or gentle back bend from lying prone

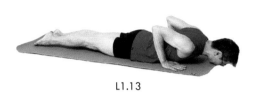

L1.13

There should be no pain in the lower back in this posture. If there is, work the tailbone in more firmly, and lengthen the ribs forward on the floor to create length in the torso. The body should be well prepared to do back bends, to avoid creating any strain; hence the spine lengthening and mobilising postures that preceded this posture in the sequence. If you find that you are getting back pain, repeat the earlier postures a few times before moving on to the next part of the sequence. Also, if you have a weakness in the lower back, you can keep the legs slightly apart in this posture.

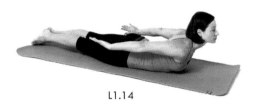

L1.14

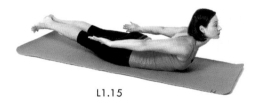

L1.15

- Lie down on your front with your forehead on the floor. Place the arms back by the hips, palms up. Move the tailbone to the floor, and reach it to your heels. Extend the ribs forward. Grip the legs together, lengthen the abdomen forward, and look forward. Broaden the collar bones, and lengthen the sides and back of your neck.

- From here, keep the tailbone pinned down, and lift the inner thighs to the ceiling, so the thighs come off the floor. Keep the legs straight, and extend the top of the feet and the toes away. At the same time, pull the arms back to the feet, and then up. Extend the chest bone and abdomen forward more.

> FOCUS ON: The engagement of the tailbone and the extension of the front body

- To come down, keep the tailbone down, lengthen the chest forward then release down to the floor, to come back to your starting position.

Makarasana

Crocodile pose, or back bend from lying prone

As with Salabhasana, there should be no pain in the lower back in this posture. If there is, work the tailbone in more firmly, and lengthen the ribs forward on the floor to create length in the torso. Also, if you have a weakness in the lower back, you can keep the legs slightly apart in this posture.

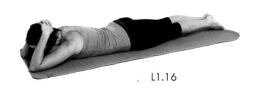

L1.16

- Lie down on your front, with the legs together. Take your hands behind the back of your head, interlacing the fingers. The thumb should catch the base of the skull. Lengthen the back of the neck away from the shoulders. Extend the side ribs forward *(L1.16)*.

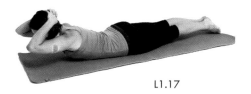

L1.17

- Grip the legs together, extend the feet away, and lift the inner thighs to the ceiling, so the thighs come off the floor. At the same time, reach the elbows strongly forward and up, and look forward. Keep the tailbone in. Reach the side ribs and the chest bone forward, and keep the top of the feet extending away *(L1.18)*.

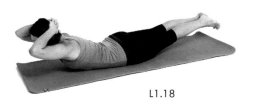

L1.18

- To come down, keep the tailbone down and extend the abdomen forward to release down.

BENEFITS:
Salabhasana and Makarasana
- Tone and strengthen the back and abdominal muscles, as well as the buttocks, backs of the legs and backs of the arms
- Open the chest and lengthen the front spine and the abdomen
- Stimulate the digestive system and the kidneys
- Relieve tension headaches and stress
- Can improve energy levels and combat low moods

L1

Bhujangasana

Snake or Cobra pose,
or backward bending from a prone position

Start by practising this pose with the forearms on the floor in front of you, to keep the action softer. Gradually, you can work towards bringing the hands back in line with the ears, and finally by the ribs. Only straighten the arms as much as is comfortable; there should never be any discomfort in the lower back. If there is stiffness or weakness in the body, it is better not to lift up too high, and to concentrate on the correct action of the tailbone, abdomen, chest and shoulders. In this way, strength and flexibility will be improved without strain or injury.

Variations

Variation 1

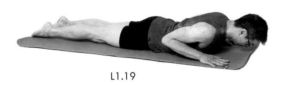

L1.19

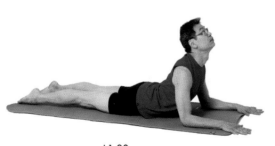

L1.20

• Lie prone, with the top of the feet on the floor, the legs together, the forehead on the floor, and the hands by the shoulders, with the fingers pointing forward. Engage the tailbone, and grip the legs together.

• Look forward, and slide the forearms forward. Press the forearms down, extend the abdomen forward, and lift and curve the chest up, broadening the collar bones *(L1.20)*. Feel that the shoulder muscles are drawn away from the ears.

• To release, keep the tailbone engaged, pull the abdomen forward to extend it back down to the floor. Rest the forehead down.

L1

Variation 2

- Place the hands by the ears. Press the hands down and look forward. Extend your pubic bone to your navel, and your navel to your chest bone. Slowly straighten the arms. As you do so, broaden the collar bones and lift the chest bone more. Draw the corners of the shoulders back. Lengthen the sides of the neck. Lift the chest more, then turn the face to look up.
- To release down, look forward. Extend the sides of the ribs forward as you lengthen back down to the mat.

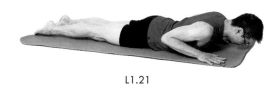

L1.21

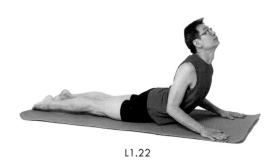

L1.22

Variation 3

- Place the hands by the side ribs, and come into the posture as you did for Variation 2. Maintain the extension and curve of the front body, then broaden and soften the back muscles.
- Release down.
- Turn the head to one side and rest it on the backs of the hands for a few moments, then change sides to rest with the head facing the other way.
- To come up, have the hands by the side ribs. Draw your abdomen strongly to your spine, and press yourself up to a kneeling position.

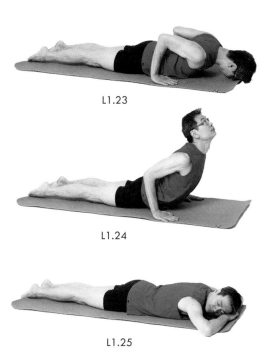

L1.23

L1.24

L1.25

L1

Urdhva Mukha Svanasana Variation

Upward facing dog, using a chair

- Be in Adho Mukha Svanasana (downward dog), with your hands on a chair or stool.

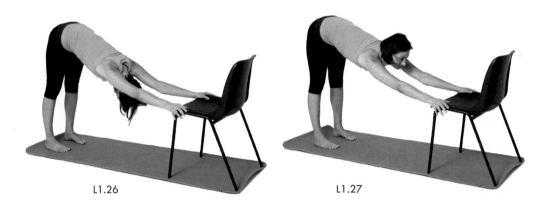

L1.26   L1.27

- Look forward. Take the weight forward into the hands. Lift your heels, press your thighs back and move your tailbone deeply in, then take your pelvis towards the chair, drawing the pubic bone to the navel at the same time. Lift the abdomen and the chest. Take the corners of the shoulders back, lift the chest more, and look up.
- To come out of this posture, look forward, suck the abdomen towards the spine and press yourself back to downward dog.
- Repeat three times.

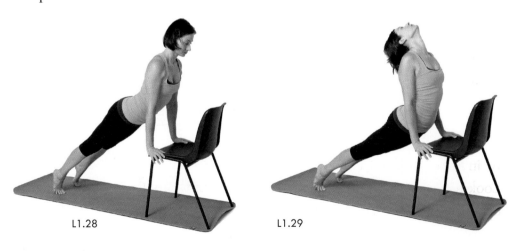

L1.28   L1.29

Urdhva Mukha Svanasana

Upward facing dog

Variations

Variation 1

- Lie down with your hands by your side ribs. Grip the legs together. Draw the elbows back to the heels, and look forward. Hold the tailbone in, and draw the top of the pubic bone forward, so the abdomen extends to the chest. Press the hands down and straighten the arms, lifting the legs and torso off the floor. Press the thighs to the ceiling, engage the tailbone in more, draw the abdomen in and up. Lift and curve the chest to the ceiling. Take the shoulders back, engage the shoulder blades in, and look up.

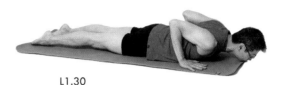

L1.30

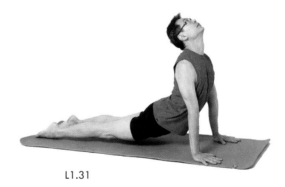

L1.31

- Look forward, and slowly release down. Bend the elbows out to the sides, and rest the head on the back of the hands.

Variation 2

- Be in Adho Mukha Svanasana.
- Look forward, then come to plank position. Lift your heels, press your thighs up and move your tailbone deeply in, then take your pelvis forward between

the arms, drawing the pubic bone to the navel at the same time *(L1.34)*. Lift the abdomen and the chest. Take the corners of the shoulders back, lift the chest more, and look up.

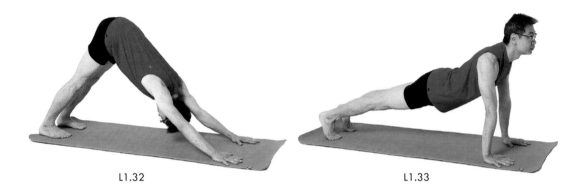

L1.32   L1.33

- To come out of this posture, look forward, suck the abdomen towards the spine and press yourself back to downward dog.

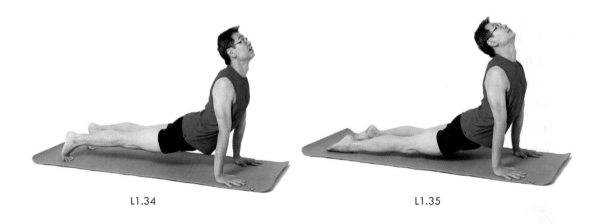

L1.34   L1.35

The next few postures are done firstly to extend the spine, then to bring it back to a neutral position after the back bends, and finally to steady the mind after the back bends, which can be very invigorating. If you choose, you can practise the upright seated postures with your back against a wall and some support behind the spine: this will make them more restful.

Baddha Konasana

Bound angle pose

If you find it difficult to lift the spine well in this posture, sit up on a support.

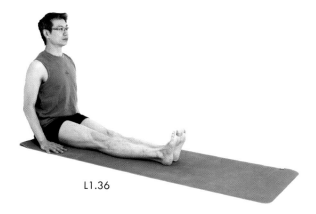

L1.36

- Sit in Dandasana. From Dandasana, come into Baddha Konasana.
- The knees should be in line with or lower than the hips, and the spine should be well lifted. Hold the feet around the toes, or hold the ankles. Hit the shin bones back towards the body, and suck the thigh bones back into the hip sockets, making the hips very firm. Feel that this helps with the lift of the spine and side trunk. Move the back armpit to the front armpit, and lift the front armpit up. Separate the collar bones, and release the shoulders away from the ears.

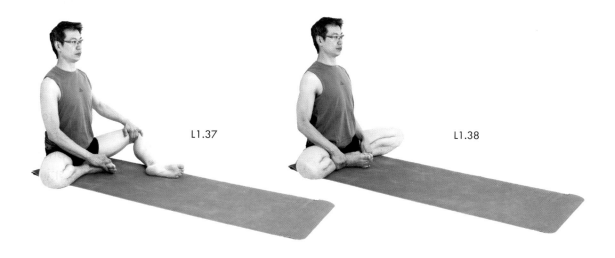

L1.37   L1.38

L1

Swastikasana, Parsva Swastikasana, then Adho Mukha Swastikasana

Sitting upright with the legs crossed, turning to the side, then going forward and resting the head

If you find it difficult to lift the spine well in this posture, sit up on a support. If you have knee problems, support the knees as shown in S3. If the ankles or feet are uncomfortable, have some padding underneath them.

Swastikasana

You may need some support for the head in the forward extension. Have a few blocks or folded blankets to hand.

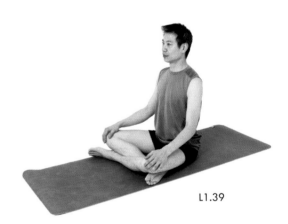

L1.39

- Sit in Dandasana. Cross the shins, so that the feet are moved well away from each other, and the knees point forward rather than out to the sides. Have a gap between the pelvis and the floor. Feel that the placement of the legs brings firmness to the hips, and allows the spine to lift.
- Lift the sides of the trunk. Release the shoulder muscles down.
- Release, and change the cross of the legs. Repeat.

Parsva Swastikasana

- Take the right hand behind you either onto the floor or onto the edge of your support. Press the hand down to lift the spine. Take the left hand onto the outer right thigh, close to the knee, and press the hand against the leg to turn the abdomen to the right. Keep the legs releasing down.
- Keep even weight on both buttock bones. Turn the abdomen, the diaphragm

and the circumference of the ribs. Move the left shoulder blade into the body to turn the chest more. Keep the collar bones lifted, and separated, and the corners of the shoulders opening back.

- Release, and change sides.
- Change the cross of the legs and repeat to both sides.

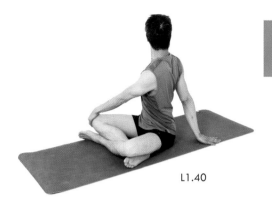

L1.40

Adho Mukha Swastikasana

- From Swastikasana, extend forward into Adho Mukha Swastikasana. From here, reach the hands forward. Keep the buttock bones pointing down. Release the head down. If your head doesn't come to the floor, place a support underneath the forehead. Rest the head and the neck.
- Come up slowly, and change sides.

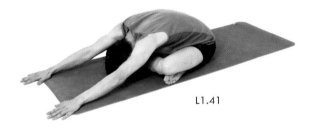

L1.41

Savasana

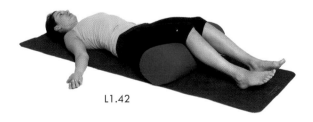

L1.42

A Quick Reminder

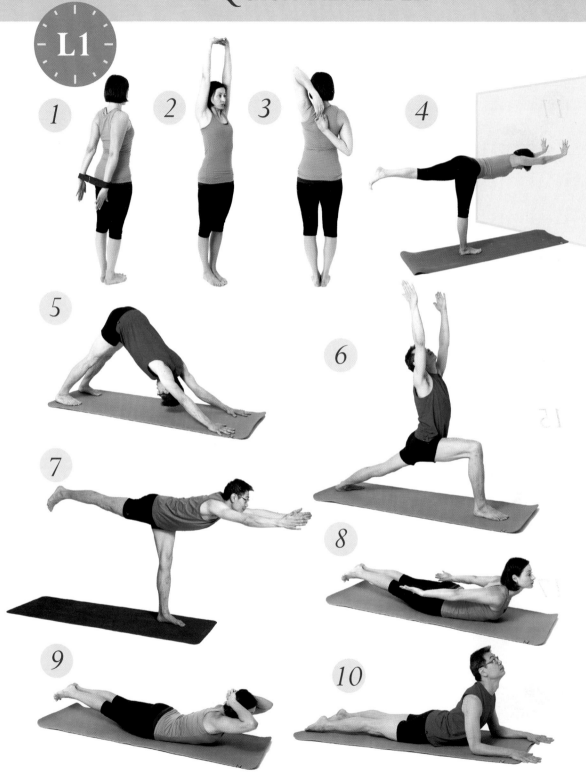

L1

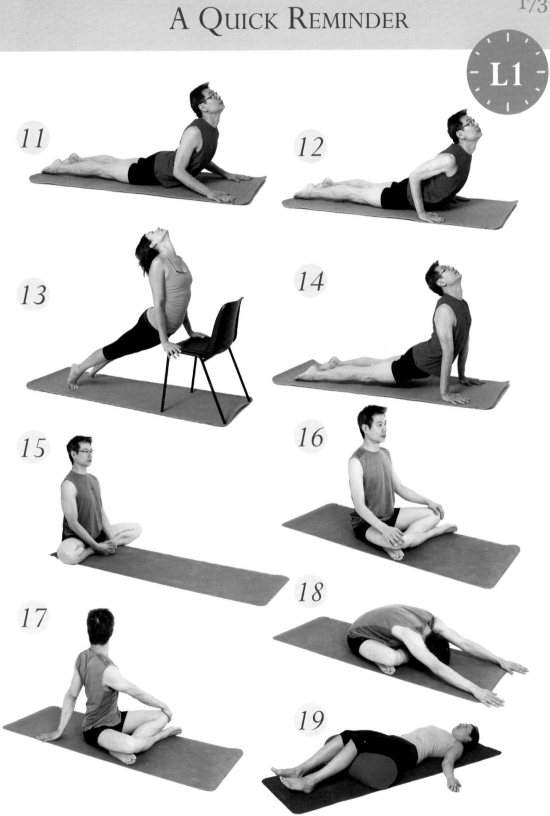

L2   LONG PROGRAMME 2

A sequence to increase the flexibility of the hips, shoulders and spine, tone the abdomen and back muscles, stimulate the digestive system and quieten the mind

YOU WILL NEED:
- A wall

YOU MAY NEED:
- A belt
- Blocks, cushions or folded towels or blankets
- A stool

Adho Mukha Virasana
and Parsva Adho Mukha Virasana

Virasana is named after a sage
Kneeling with the head down forward, then to the side

- Be in Adho Mukha Virasana, with the knees hip bone width apart, and the big toes just touching each other. Extend the arms.
- Reach the buttock bones and tailbone down, and lengthen the sides of the body forward.
- Come into Parsva Adho Mukha Virasana, turning to the right first. Extend the left hand away. Pin the left buttock bone down, so that there is full extension on the left side of the body. Turn the abdomen to the right. Keep the back body broad as you turn.

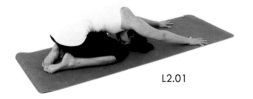

L2.01

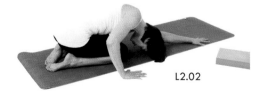

L2.02

- Move the hands back to their original positions and bring yourself back to centre. Change sides.

Swastikasana and Parsva Swastikasana

Sitting upright with the legs crossed, then turning to the side

- Sit in Swastikasana with the right leg in front.
- Lift the sides of the body up. Lift the front armpit chest. Broaden the collar bones. Lift the back ribs, but keep the skin of the back body releasing down.
- Release and change sides.

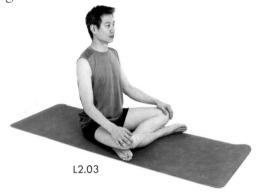

L2.03

Parsva Swastikasana

- Come into Parsva Swastikasana, turning to the right first. Lift and broaden the collar bones. Lift the back ribs, but keep the shoulder muscles releasing down. Let the head follow the turn of the spine.
- Keep even weight on both buttock bones. Open the corners of the shoulders back.
- Release, and change sides.
- Change the cross of the legs and repeat.

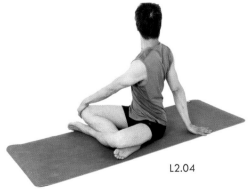

L2.04

L2

Adho Mukha Svanasana

Downward facing dog

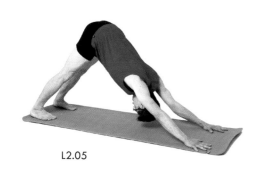

L2.05

- Be in Adho Mukha Svanasana. Lift the kneecaps well, and move the top of the knees back. Reach the lower part of the calf muscle down to the heel, and press the centre of the back of the heel down into or towards the floor. Lengthen the sole of the foot from the ball of the foot to the heel.
- Lengthen the skin on the back of the head to the crown of the head. Feel that the spine is extending fully.

Uttanasana

Intense stretch pose

- Be in Uttanasana.
- Grip the outer ankles in, and lift the inner ankles, inner knees and inner thighs up. Draw the lower abdomen in, and reach the chest bone and the front armpits to the floor, lifting the back thighs and the buttock bones up more. Take the weight into the back of the balls of the feet, broaden the backs of the legs, and

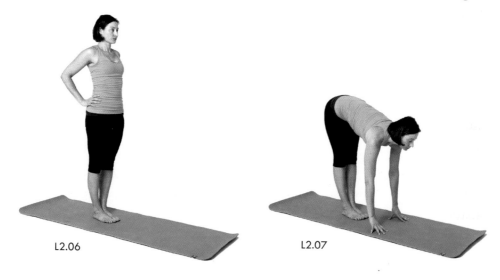

L2.06   L2.07

lift and separate the buttock bones. Bend the elbows back, and draw the sides of the body down to the floor and in to the legs.

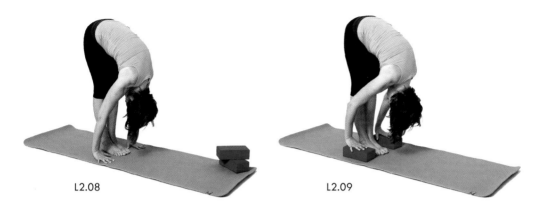

L2.08   L2.09

Uttanasana Variation

Intense stretch pose, with the back to a wall

If you are stiff in the hamstrings or the back, you'll need to start with the feet further away from the wall – try this once or twice until you get the right distance. Don't twist as you come into this posture or come out of it – bend the knees and use the hands against the wall instead to come into it without twisting the spine.

- Come into Uttanasana with your back against the wall *(L2.13)*. Press the big toe joints down, extend the soles of the feet back, and pin the heel bones down. Open the backs of the knees, lift the back thighs, and keep the front thigh muscles lifting strongly.
- To come up, place your hands on the floor and take the weight into the hands. Bend the knees, and walk your hands up the wall to push yourself up. Bend the knees more, bring your head up, and come back to a standing position.

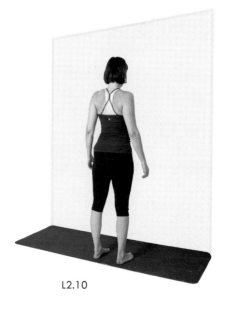

L2.10

L2

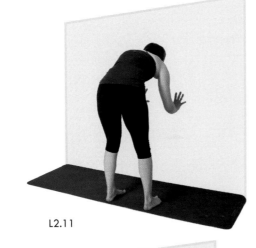

L2.11

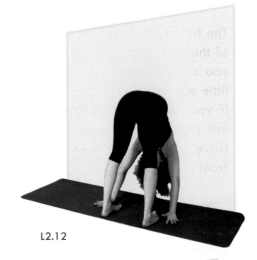

L2.12

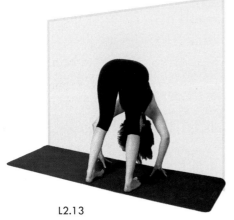

L2.13

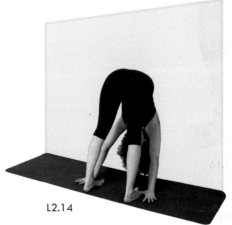

L2.14

BENEFITS:
Uttanasana
- Strengthens the legs
- Improves flexibility in the hamstrings
- Creates flexibility and reduces tension in the lower back
- Brings quietness to the mind

Parsvottanasana

Intense stretch posture to the side,
or a standing extension for the spine

If you like, you can do this once using a chair, as you have practised in S4, then try the full posture.

The front foot should be in line with the instep of the back foot in this posture, but if you find you can't balance like this, take the feet a little wider.

If you can't reach the floor with the hands in this posture, take support under the hands. Have two blocks or bricks ready towards the front (narrow) edge of your mat.

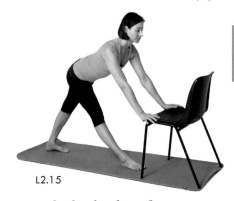

L2.15

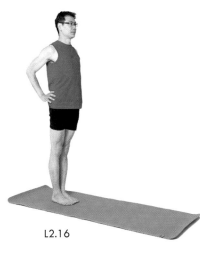

L2.16

• Stand in Tadasana at the back edge of your mat. Come into Parsvottanasana extending forward, with the right leg in front. Press the back heel down, and lift the arch of the foot. Press the front big toe joint down, and lift the shin bone and thigh up. Extend the front body forward. Reach the pubic bone to the navel, the navel to the chest bone and the chest bone to the chin.

• From here, bend the elbows back to reach the chest bone towards your front leg. Let the head and neck release *(L2.20)*.

• To come out of this posture, look forward, place the fingertips on the hips and lift the thighs muscles and abdomen strongly, then extend the chest bone forward and up. Bend the legs and step forward to release, then come back to your starting position to do the other side.

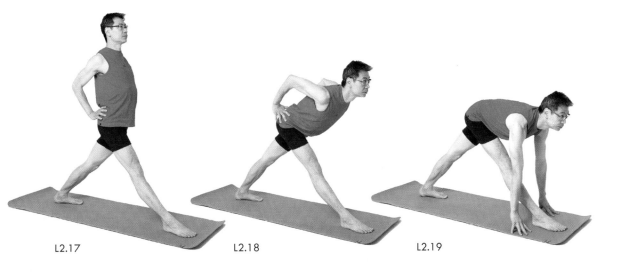

L2.17   L2.18   L2.19

L2

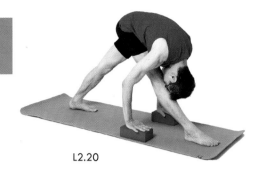

L2.20

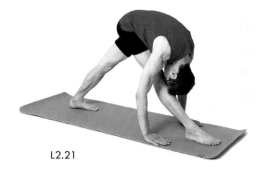

L2.21

Marichyasana 1, as a forward bend

Marichyasana is named after a sage
Forward bend, with one leg bent

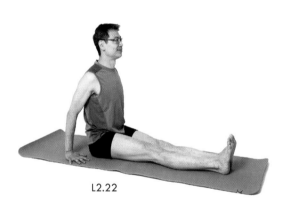

L2.22

• Sit in Dandasana. Bend your right leg, so that the heel is in line with its own buttock bone. Clasp the shin and lift the spine well. Extend the left foot away, but draw the left thigh bone firmly back into the hip socket.

• Reach the right hand up, draw the lower abdomen in and up, and extend the chest forward towards the left toes. Take the right arm in front of the right shin, turn the palm to face behind you, then bend the arm to reach the hand back behind the sacrum. Extend the left arm out and back to catch the hands. If you can't quite reach, take a belt in the left hand and gently swing it to catch it with the

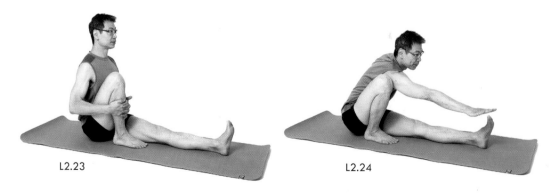

L2.23

L2.24

right fingers. Pull the hands together, and feel that the right shin hits back, allowing you to lengthen the chest and front armpits forward more *(L2.25)*. Rest the head down *(L2.26)*.

• Release, come back to Dandasana, and change sides.

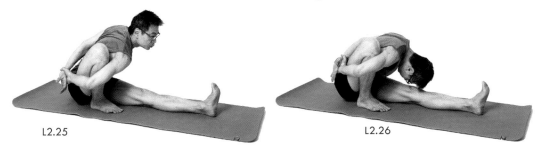

L2.25   L2.26

Paschimottanasana, going forward, then resting the head

Intense stretch of the back body, or seated forward bend

If there is stiffness in the legs, hips or spine, and you feel that going forward is impossible, try having the feet hip width apart instead of together. If you find it challenging to sit with the legs straight and the front body lifted in Dandasana, sit up on a support.

If you can't hold the feet in this posture, place a belt around the balls of the feet instead, holding it with the hands shoulder width apart *(L2.28)*. In this position, concentrate on the extension of the spine, rather than trying to take the head down.

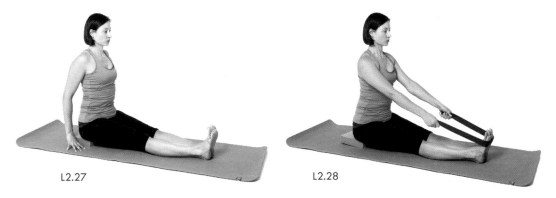

L2.27   L2.28

• Sit in Dandasana. Grip the hips in, and lift the sides of the body up. Extend

L2

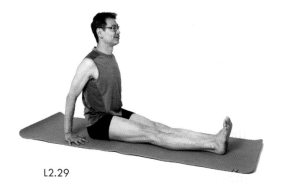

L2.29

the inner balls of the feet and the inner heels away, but draw the thigh muscles towards the body, and press them down. Feel that the front body is well lifted.

- Extend the chest bone forward, hinging from the hips. Hold the outside edges of the feet with the hands *(L2.30)*. Reach the backs of the legs back. Pull on the feet, but resist the balls of the feet away. Bend the elbows out, and extend the sides of the body forward. Let the head rest down *(L2.31)*.

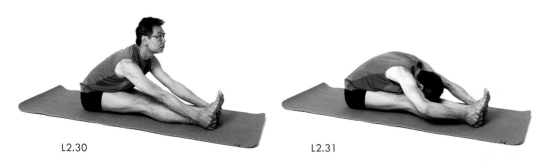

L2.30   L2.31

Upavistha Konasana, with variations (Parsva, then forward)

Seated angle pose, upright, then to the side, then forward

- Sit in Dandasana. Press the fingertips down into the floor on either side of your hips, grip your hips together and lift the sides of the body up.
- Feel that you are sitting on the very centre of the top of the sitting bones. The balls of the feet reach away, and the thigh muscles and the bones of the thighs move back into the hip sockets, aiding the lift of the spine. Without disturbing the alignment, take the legs as wide as you comfortably can. The toes should continue to point at the ceiling – don't let them roll out. Keep the buttock bones pinned down, the thighs active and the front spine lifted.

Upavistha Konasana with Urdhva Hastasana

- Stretch the arms up, keeping the hands shoulder width apart. Have the palms facing each other *(L2.32)*. Reach into the wrists and fingers, keeping the shoulders away from the ears. Move the inner thighs down. Keep the lift of the sides of the body as you take the arms back down.

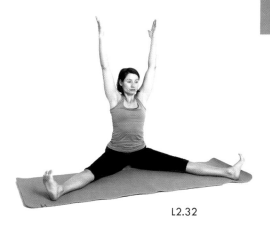

L2.32

Variations

Parsva Upavistha Konasana

- Pin the left buttock bone down, and turn your abdomen towards your right thigh. Keep the front spine ascending. Place the hands on either side of the right thigh, and use the hands on the floor to turn the abdomen more. Keep the chest lifted. Turn the diaphragm to the right. Turn the circumference of the ribs. Only turn the head when the rest of the spine is fully turned. Keep the left buttock bone pinned firmly down. Look forward, and release. Change sides.

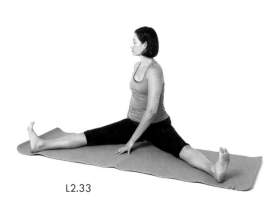

L2.33

Forward Variation 1

- Pin the inner and outer thighs down. Without disturbing the legs, take the hands forward between the legs, and reach the chest forward *(L2.35)*. Lengthen the chest and the abdomen forward. Keep the shoulders away from the ears.

L2

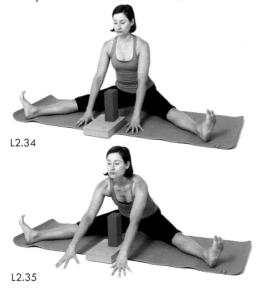

L2.34

Finally, rest the head down. If the head doesn't reach the floor, take as much support as is needed to let the forehead rest down *(L2.36)*.

L2.35

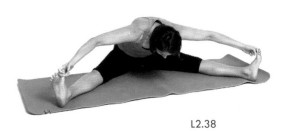

L2.36

Forward Variation 2

- Take the big toes with the index finger and middle finger of each hand, with the palms facing in *(L2.37)*. If this isn't possible, take a belt over the ball of each foot *(L2.39)*. Pull on the toes or the belt, but at the same time extend the feet away. Take the chest forward. When the front spine is fully extended, bend the elbows out to the sides, and lengthen the side ribs forward more.

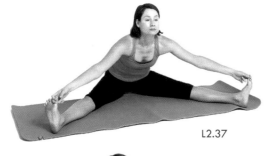

L2.37

L2.38

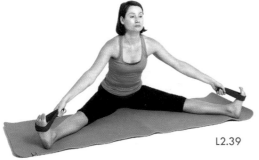

L2.39

There should be no pain in the backs of the knees in this posture. If there is, it is a sign that the muscles of the legs aren't working correctly, or the feet and legs aren't correctly placed. The inner edges of the balls of the feet and the heels should reach away strongly. The front thighs and all four corners of the knees should stay facing upward.

Resting Variation

- Have a long support – a bolster, or blocks, or folded blankets – between the legs, in front of your abdomen *(L2.40)*. Sit up well, and draw the support in towards you so that it touches your pelvis. Lift the abdomen up, and lengthen the chest forward to place the abdomen onto the bolster.

- Feel that you have placed yourself so you can support the whole of the abdomen and the front chest on the bolster. Rest the back body down. You can rest the forehead down, or rest turning the head to one side.

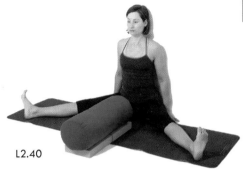

L2.40

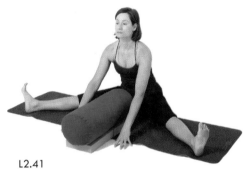

L2.41

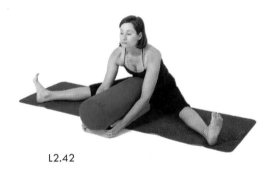

L2.42

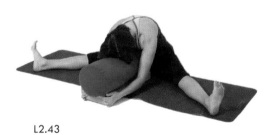

L2.43

Savasana

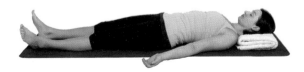

L2.44

A QUICK REMINDER

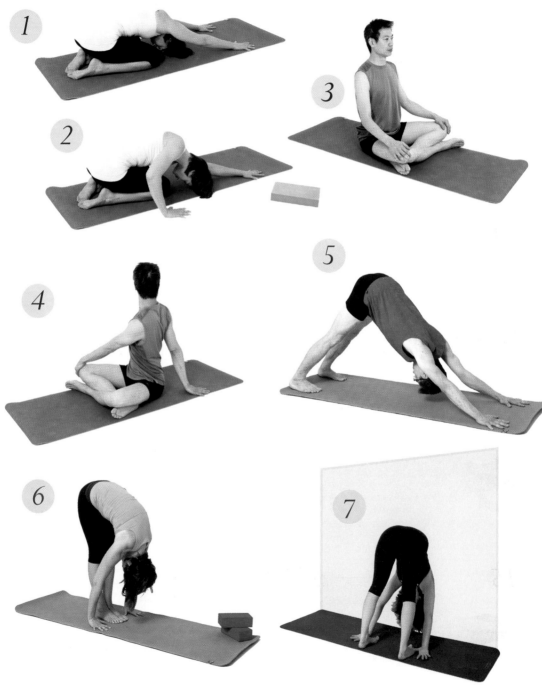

1

2

3

4

5

6

7

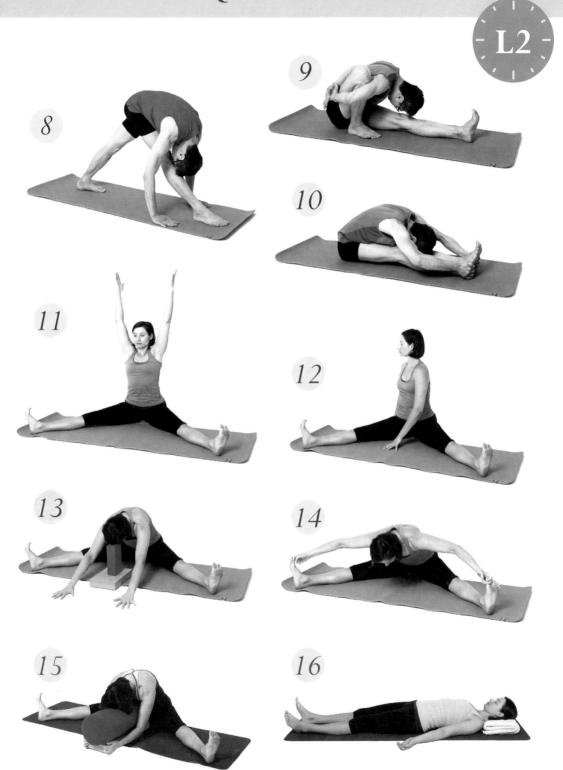

L2

8

9

10

11

12

13

14

15

16

L3 | LONG PROGRAMME 3

A sequence to increase the flexibility of the hips, ankles and shoulders, lengthen the spine and abdomen, stimulate the digestive system and open the chest. Many of the postures given here can be practised with support in order to create a recuperative sequence. Because of this, fewer asanas are given, so that more time can be spent on each.

YOU MAY NEED:
- A belt
- Blocks, cushions or folded towels or blankets

Supta Baddha Konasana

Supine bound angle pose

If you wish to make this a restful practice, place support under the back, as shown for supported Savasana on page 26, and also under the outer legs, as shown in Supta Swastikasana later in this sequence. Take support under the back of the head and neck if appropriate. Skip the arm variations so you can completely relax into the posture.

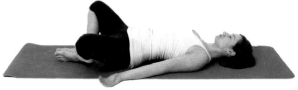

L3.01

- Lie down in Supta Baddha Konasana *(L3.01)*.
- Release the shoulder muscles away from the ears, and engage the back ribs up. Lengthen the flesh of the buttocks to the heels. Feel that the sacrum is moving lightly up into the body, allowing the legs to release down. Lengthen the skin

on the back of the head away from the shoulders, and soften the skin on the forehead down towards the eyebrows, and out to the temples. When you have made all these adjustments, relax. Soften and broaden the abdomen. Relax the back. Soften the jaw.

Arm Variations

Variation 1

- Stretch your hands to the ceiling, with the palms facing each other, about shoulder width apart *(L3.02)*. Keep the tailbone lengthening towards the heels. Extend your fingers to the floor behind your head *(L3.04)*. If the hands don't reach all the way to the floor, place a cushion or other support underneath them, so that you can rest them down. Lengthen your fingers away from the shoulders, but at the same time draw the shoulders away from your ears.

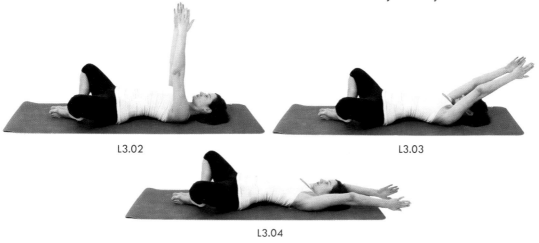

L3.02

L3.03

L3.04

Variation 2

- Clasp your elbows above your chest *(L3.05)*. Reach the elbows towards the floor behind your head. If the elbows don't reach all the way to the floor, place a cushion or other support underneath them, so you can rest them down *(L3.06)*. Keep the shoulders away from the ears, and the elbows reaching away. Release, change the cross of the forearms, and repeat on the other side.

L3

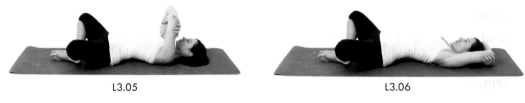

L3.05   L3.06

Variation 3

- Interlace your fingers together. Turn the palms to the ceiling, press the fingers into the backs of the hands *(L3.07)*, then take the hands towards the floor behind your head. Keep the shoulders extending away from the ears *(L3.08)*. Press the fingers away firmly to open the palms of the hands. Release, change the interlacing of the fingers, so that the other thumb is on top, and repeat.

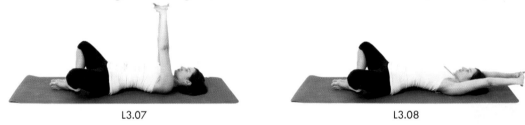

L3.07   L3.08

Virasana with Garudasana and Urdhva Baddhanguliyasana

Kneeling posture, with arm variations
(Eagle and upward bound fingers positions)

If you wish you make this a restful practice, have some padding under your legs, so that you can sit without discomfort. Sit up on a support to assist with the lift of the spine. Skip the arm variations, and just sit quietly.

- Sit in Virasana *(L3.09)*.
- Lift the abdominal muscles up and soften them back. Lift the chest bone. Feel that the back of the head is in line with the back of the sacrum.
- Take the palms of the hands onto the soles

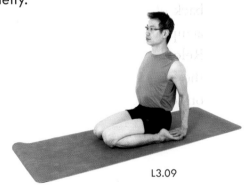

L3.09

of the feet, with the fingers pointing to the heels, and the base of the hands in contact with the toes. Stretch the skin of the palms of the hands to the fingers, and press the hands down to lift the sides of the body up more. Move the back armpit to the front armpit, and lift the front armpit to the ceiling.

Arm Variations

Garudasana

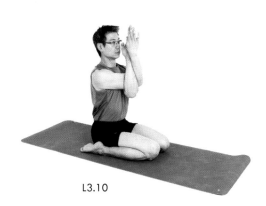

L3.10

- Bring the arms into Garudasana, with the right arm underneath first. Lift the chest bone up, then lift your elbows up off your chest. Move the hands away from your face. Keep your collar bones lifted and separated, and the muscles of the shoulders releasing down the back.
- Release and change the cross of the arms.

Urdhva Baddhanguliyasana

- Bring the hands into Urdhva Baddhanguliyasana. Keep the shoulders away from the ears, and the abdomen moving back, and lifting up. Move the back of the armpit to the front of the armpit, and lift the front armpit up.
- Release, then change the interlacing of the fingers, so that the other thumb is on top, and repeat.

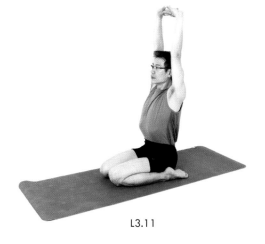

L3.11

Supta Virasana, with or without support

L3

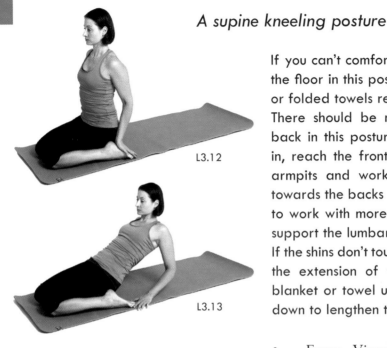

L3.12

L3.13

A *supine kneeling posture*

If you can't comfortably take your back on to the floor in this posture, have a bolster, blocks or folded towels ready to use as support.

There should be no discomfort in the lower back in this posture. If there is, grip the hips in, reach the frontal hip bones towards your armpits and work the tailbone more firmly towards the backs of the knees. You may need to work with more support under the back to support the lumbar.

If the shins don't touch the floor, this can hamper the extension of the spine. Place a folded blanket or towel under the shins. Pin the shins down to lengthen the spine out of the pelvis.

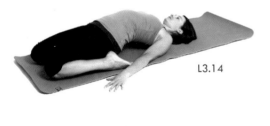

L3.14

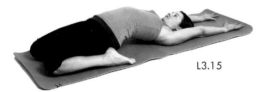

L3.15

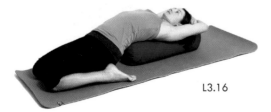

L3.16

• From Virasana *(L3.12)*, come into Supta Virasana *(L3.14)*. Grip the hips in and lengthen the tailbone towards the backs of the knees. Draw the frontal hip bones to your armpits. Reach the arms over the head and take the hands to the floor, with the palms facing up *(L3.15)*, and the hands shoulder width apart – or, if you are on a support, clasp the elbows behind your head *(L3.16)*. Reach the hands or elbows away to extend the body more, but keep the upper arm bones moving back into the shoulder sockets, so there is a firmness on the outer shoulders, which mirrors the firmness on the outer hips.

• To come up, take the hands to the feet. Press the elbows into the floor to lift yourself up.

Variation on Setu Bandha Sarvangasana, with support

L3

Bridge posture,
which when done with support is a supine front-opening pose

If you are fairly stiff in the spine or shoulders, or have back problems, have a low support under your pelvis. If you are quite flexible, have a higher support.
If you are doing this as a resting posture, practise this with a soft support under the pelvis – such as a cushion or bolster – and make sure it is not too high.

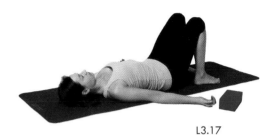

L3.17

- Lie down with the knees bent and the feet on the floor *(L3.17)*. Lift the hips and place your support centrally under the sacrum *(L3.18)*. Rotate the upper arms from the inside to the outside, so that the armpits open. Engage the shoulder blades and dorsal spine up into the body so the chest opens *(L3.19)*. Keep the flesh of the buttocks moving to the heels, extend the legs away one at a time. Move your inner thighs down, and reach the balls of the feet away. Broaden and soften the abdomen. Broaden the back muscles *(L3.20)*.

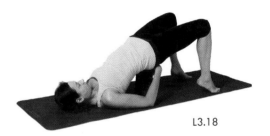

L3.18

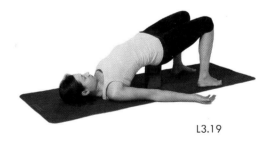

L3.19

- To release, bend your legs, and bring the soles of the feet to the floor. Lift your pelvis, and remove the support. Lengthen the spine slowly down, pulling the tailbone to your heels as you do so. Roll on to your side to come up.

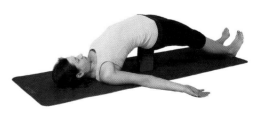

L3.20

L3

BENEFITS:

Setu Bandha Sarvangasana
- Relieves menstrual discomfort and abdominal irritation
- Opens the chest and pelvis
- Improves flexibility in the spine, shoulders and hips
- Lengthens the abdomen and front spine, allowing the lungs and digestive organs to work more efficiently
- Tones the back muscles
- Brings quietness to the mind

Swastikasana

Cross-legged seated position

The knees should be in line with or lower than the hips, and the spine should be well lifted. If you find that the legs are lifting or the back dropping, sit up on a support. If the knees, ankles or feet are uncomfortable, have some padding underneath them.

- Sit in Swastikasana. Broaden the buttock crease from the inside to the outside and engage the sacrum in, so you are sitting right on the top of the buttock bones.
- Draw the lower abdomen gently in, and lift the chest bone up. Feel that the thigh bones rotate in the hip sockets from the inside to the outside, and the outer thighs extend from the hips to the outer knees, to bring the legs in towards each other.
- Release and change sides.

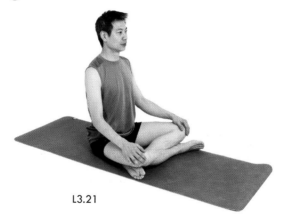

L3.21

Supta Swastikasana

Supine cross-legged pose

If you are doing this as a resting posture, or if there is any strain in the knees or pelvis in Supta Swastikasana, take support under the thighs and knees, so that you can allow the legs to release down fully.

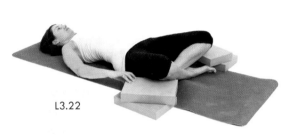

L3.22

- Sit in Swastikasana.
- Grip the hips in, and take the hands back behind the hips. Bend the elbows one at a time, and take the elbows to the floor. Lengthen the sides of the body away from the pelvis, and reach the tailbone to the heels. Finally take the shoulders to the floor, reaching the muscles of the shoulders away from the ears.
- Lengthen the top buttock and the back of the tailbone to the feet. Engage the sacrum up into the body lightly – without letting the abdomen or lumbar lift. Feel that this action allows the knees to release down to the floor, which will encourage the pelvis to open, and the abdomen to lengthen and broaden.
- Reach the hands over the head, palms facing up *(L3.23)*. Lengthen the fingers away, but keep the bones of the upper arms moving back into the shoulder sockets, and the back armpit moving to the front armpit.

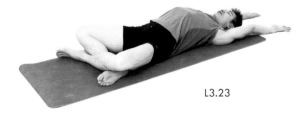

L3.23

- To change sides, unfold the legs, and bring the soles of the feet to the floor. Change the cross of the legs without disturbing the rest of the body. To ensure you work the body evenly, start on the second side the next time you practise this posture.

Supta Tadasana

Supine mountain pose

If you are practising this as resting posture, take support under the back body and head, as shown for supported Savasana on page 26. You can miss out the arm variations.

- Lie down, with the knees bent, and the soles of the feet on the floor. Move the shoulder muscles away from the ears. Scrub the heels away from you on the floor one at a time; feel that this makes the legs very active. Move the front thigh muscles down to hold the bones of the thighs. Reach the flesh of the top buttocks and the skin and flesh of the sacrum to the heels. Extend the inner ankles away.

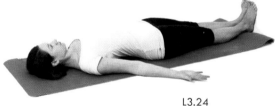

L3.24

Arm Variations

Variation 1

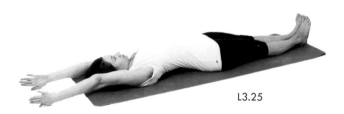

L3.25

- Stretch your fingers to the floor behind your head, with the palms facing each other, shoulder width apart.

Variation 2

- Clasp the elbows behind your head. Draw the corners of the elbows away from you, but keep the shoulders moving away from the ears. Engage the shoulder blades up towards the chest, and feel the elbows release down more. Move the tailbone to the heels, and feel that the abdomen releases down to the spine.

- Release, change the cross of the forearms, and repeat on the other side.

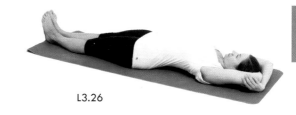

L3.26

Variation 3

- With the fingers interlaced, take the hands towards the floor behind your head. Extend the thumb side of the hands away more. Draw the pubic bone to the navel, the navel to the chest bone, and the chest bone to the chin.
- Release, change the interlacing of the fingers, so that the other thumb is on top, and repeat.

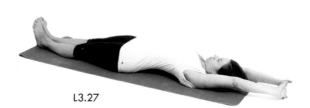

L3.27

Savasana

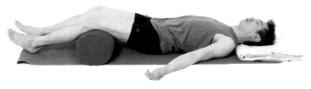

L3.28

A QUICK REMINDER

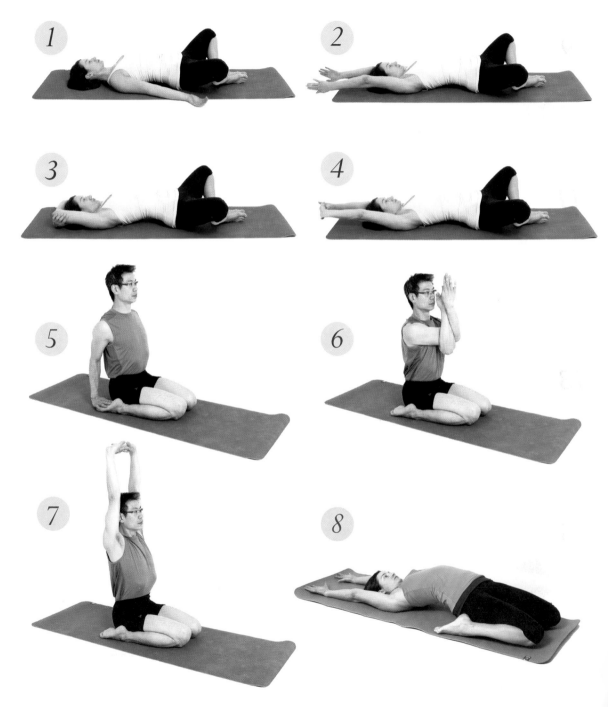

9

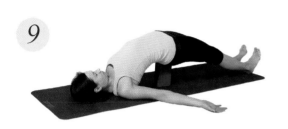

10

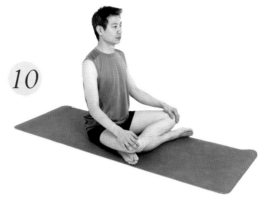

11

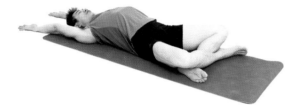

12

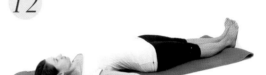

13

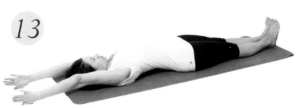

14

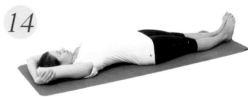

15

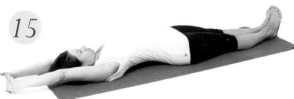

16

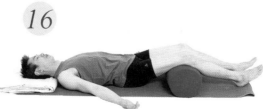

L4   LONG PROGRAMME 4

A sequence to increase the flexibility of the hips, shoulders and spine, tone the abdomen and back muscles and stimulate the digestive system

YOU WILL NEED:
- A wall
- A belt
- A block

YOU MAY NEED:
- Blocks, cushions or folded towels or blankets

Viparita Karani

Inverse action posture

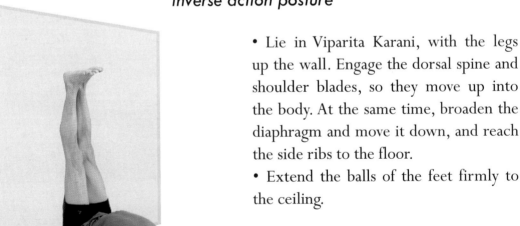

L4.01

- Lie in Viparita Karani, with the legs up the wall. Engage the dorsal spine and shoulder blades, so they move up into the body. At the same time, broaden the diaphragm and move it down, and reach the side ribs to the floor.
- Extend the balls of the feet firmly to the ceiling.

Adho Mukha Svanasana Variation

Downward facing dog pose, with the heels on a wall

L4

- Place your mat so that the short edge touches a wall, then kneel down so that your toes are close to, but not touching, the wall. Place the hands shoulder width apart, with the wrists further forward than the shoulders *(L4.02)*.

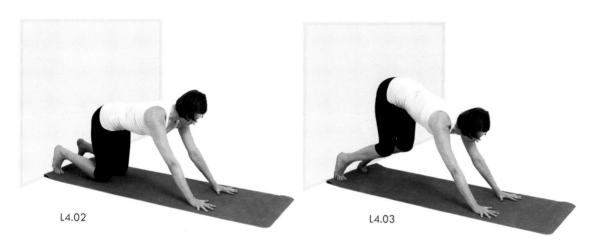

L4.02   L4.03

- Now tuck your toes under, lift your hips up and straighten the legs so that the heels press into the wall *(L4.05)*. Feel that this action allows you to work the top of the thighs back more firmly, and engage the shoulder blades more deeply towards the shins.

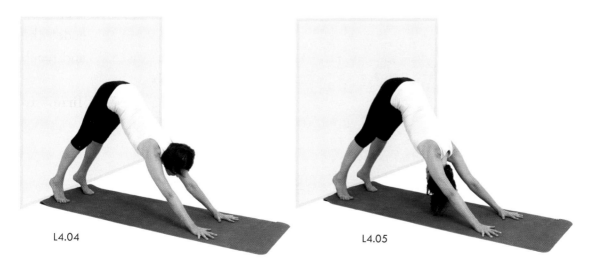

L4.04   L4.05

Preparation for Virabhadrasana 1

Warrior 1

• Be in Adho Mukha Svanasana, with the heels on the wall, as above.

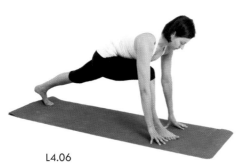

L4.06

• Look forward, and step your right foot centrally between your hands. Have the ankle under the knee. Press the back heel into the wall firmly, and draw the right hip back, so there is even length on both sides of the body *(L4.06)*. Move your tailbone in. Reach your chest bone forward.

• Step the front foot back to return to downward dog. Repeat on the other side.

Parivrtta Parsvakonasana Variation

Revolved side angle pose, with the back heel to the wall

You may need some support for the lower hand in this posture. Have a block ready towards the front right edge of your mat.

The final position can be quite challenging, so it has been split into stages so that you can progress gradually to the final posture. Make sure one stage is coming well before you proceed to the next stage, so that you maintain good alignment in the posture, and don't strain yourself.

• Be in the Virabhadrasana 1 preparatory posture, as above, with the right leg forward *(L4.06)*.

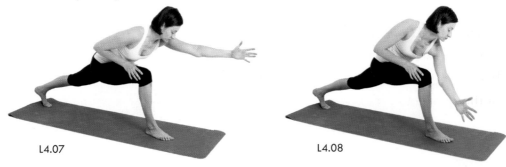

L4.07   L4.08

- Keep the back heel pressing into the wall, and the front thigh muscle lifting up to hold the thigh bone. Reach the left arm forward, then across to the outside of the right leg *(L4.09)*. Bend the elbow towards its opposite hip, and reach your outer shoulder to the outside of the thigh. Straighten the arm so that the hand reaches to the floor *(L4.10)*. If you can't reach the floor, take your hand onto your support.

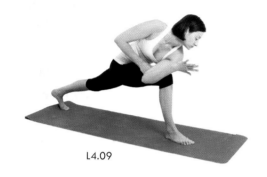

L4.09

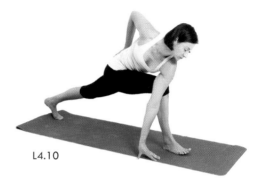

L4.10

Stage 1

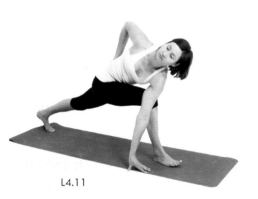

L4.11

- Take the right hand to the sacrum, and open the top shoulder to the ceiling. Using your arm against the bent leg, turn the whole of the abdomen as if you were trying to take it through the gap between the leg and body. Keep the back leg firm, the right outer hip extending back, and the tailbone in.

Stage 2

- Stretch the back arm up to the ceiling. Press the lower arm against the bent leg and the bent leg against the arm to increase the turn of the spine and torso.

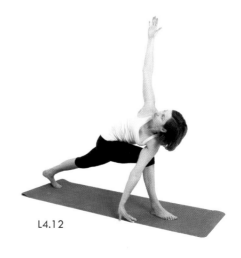

L4.12

Stage 3

- Turn the chest more towards the ceiling, then reach the upper arm towards your upper ear, so that it points diagonally away from your back heel. Keep the shoulder away from the ear, extend the fingers away, and lengthen the right outer hip back. Turn the abdomen more.

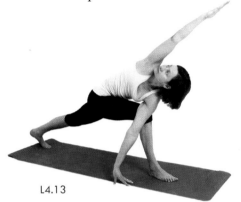

L4.13

- Slowly release, place the hands on either side of the front foot and extend the spine forward, then step back to downward dog and change sides.

> FOCUS ON: Drawing the front outer hip back, to keep the sides of the body lengthening

Preparation for Pincha Mayurasana

Preparation for feathered peacock pose, or elbow or forearm balance

When done as a preparatory pose, this posture works the shoulders strongly, opening the chest and armpits.

- Have a belt with a loop in it that is as wide as your shoulders, and a block. Place the belt around your elbows, making sure that the buckle doesn't touch the flesh. Kneel, with your forearms on the floor. Place the block between your wrists – this is to keep the wrists aligned with the shoulders.

Variations

Variation 1

- Turn your palms up, and stretch your thumbs to the floor. Feel that the inner upper arms rotate from the inside to the outside. Tuck your toes under, lift your hips and move your thighs back – as if you were doing downward dog with your legs and torso. Look in between the arms, and press the backs of the hands down to move the shoulder blades in to the body.

* Release back down to your kneeling position.

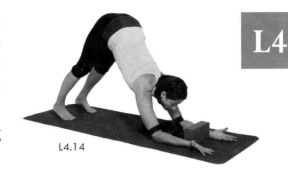

L4.14

Variation 2

* Turn the hands so that the palms face each other – but keep the rotation of the upper arms. Repeat as above. Keep the inner upper arms rotating strongly from the inside to the outside, and press the shoulder blades into the body. Suck the lower abdomen to the spine, and press the outer hips back.
* Release back down to your kneeling position.

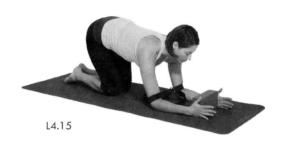

L4.15

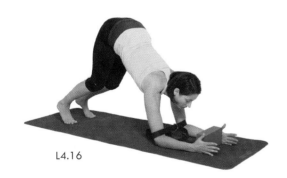

L4.16

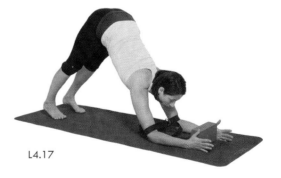

L4.17

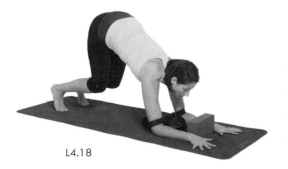

L4.18

Variation 3

* Keep the rotation of the inner upper arms from the inside to the outside, and turn the palms to the floor. Without disturbing the upper arms, pin the inner

L4

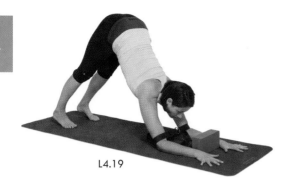

L4.19

wrists down. Repeat as above. Keep the inner upper arms lifting up, and the shoulders lifting up, away from the ears. Keep the diaphragm drawn into the body, and broad. Press the top of the thighs back.

• Release.

Urdhva Prasarita Padasana

Upward extended feet pose, or lying supine with the legs raised

If you have a back problem, only practise Variation 1, and keep the hands by the hips, with the palms down.

• Lie in Supta Tadasana. Lengthen the tailbone to the heels, so the abdomen moves down. Stretch the arms over the head. Bend the knees *(L4.20)*.

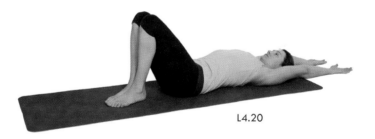

L4.20

Variations

Variation 1

• Bend the knees into the chest *(L4.21)*, then stretch the legs to the ceiling. Extend the fingers away, and keep the balls of the feet reaching up. Hold the abdomen to the spine, but keep the abdomen and the front of the pelvis broad *(L4.22)*.
• Bend the knees, and release the feet to the floor.
• Repeat twice.

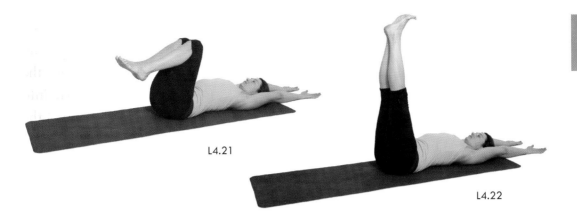

L4.21

L4.22

Variation 2

- Bend the knees into the chest, then stretch the legs to the ceiling. Extend the fingers away more, and keep the balls of the feet reaching up. Hold the abdomen down to the spine, and broaden the diaphragm. Keep the arms extending and the abdomen moving firmly down, and slowly bring the legs down to a sixty degree position *(L4.23)*. Hold here for a few moments, then bring the legs down to a thirty degree position *(L4.24)*. Hold here for a few moments, then bring the legs down so the feet hover just off the floor *(L4.25)*. Finally, release the feet down. Repeat twice.

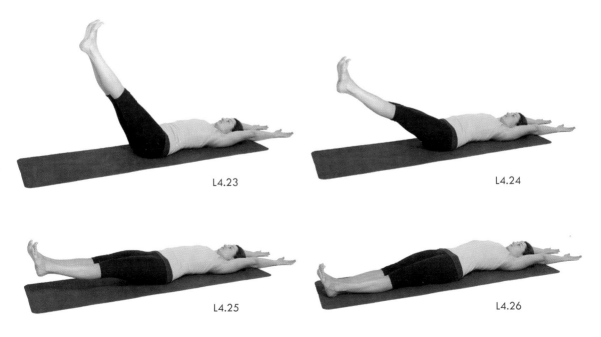

L4.23

L4.24

L4.25

L4.26

L4

Ardha Navasana

Half boat posture,
or balancing seated posture raising both legs

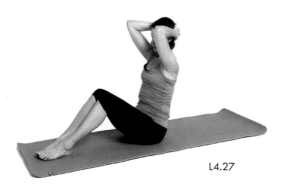

L4.27

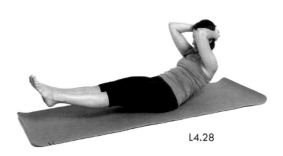

L4.28

- Sit in Dandasana, and clasp the hands behind the head. The thumbs should just sit in the base of the skull. Lengthen the base of the skull away from the shoulders, but keep the chest bone well lifted. The elbows reach forward, and up, encouraging the lift of the side ribs and chest.

- Keep the diaphragm drawing back, and slowly recline the body until the top and back of the buttocks are on the floor *(L4.27)*. Keep the gaze forward, at eye level. From here, raise the legs until the toes come to the same height as your eyes. Reach the balls of the feet away, but draw the thighs firmly back towards the hips *(L4.28)*.

- To come up, lift from the chest bone to pull yourself back to vertical.

Paripurna Navasana

Full boat pose, or balancing seated position raising the legs high

- Sit in Dandasana. Draw the abdomen back to the spine, and engage the sacrum into the body. Reach the inner edges of the feet away, but draw the thighs back towards the hips. Grip the legs together *(L4.29)*.

- From here, lift the legs up until the feet are in line with the knees, and at the same time, recline a little way back – but not as far as in Ardha Navasana. Feel that you are balancing on the top of the buttock bones, and the lower back and abdomen are lifting strongly. Straighten your legs, so the toes are higher than the top of your head. Stretch the arms out at shoulder height, with the palms facing each other (*L4.31*).

- To come up, lift the chest bone, release the legs down and come back to Dandasana.
- If you choose, you can try going from Paripurna Navasana to Ardha Navasana, and back up to Paripurna Navasana – this is a strong abdominal workout. Repeat several times, moving with control and steadiness.

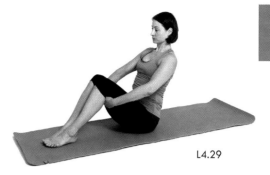

L4.29

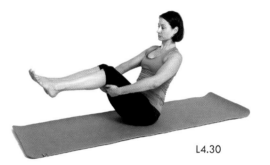

L4.30

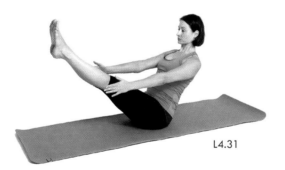

L4.31

BENEFITS:
Ardha Navasana and Paripurna Navasana
- Strengthens and tones the back and abdominal muscles, and the hip flexors
- Tones the legs and arms
- Improves flexibility in the hips and sacrum
- Improves focus and discipline in the practice

L4

Jathara Parivartanasana, in two ways

Revolved abdomen pose

- Lie down on your back, with the knees bent, and the arms extended to the sides *(L4.32)*.

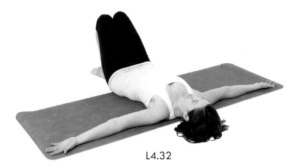

L4.32

Pawanmuktasana

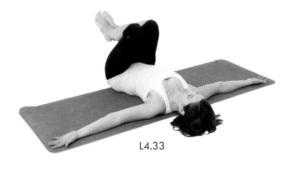

L4.33

- Bring the knees in towards the chest. Hold the legs together. Draw the inner thighs to the groins. Pull the toes in towards the shins, and press the heels away. Broaden the abdomen and the front pelvis *(L4.33)*.

Variations

Jathara Parivartanasana, with legs bent

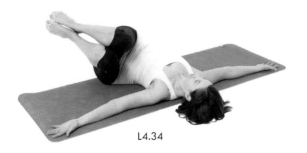

L4.34

- Extend the fingers away from each other. Grip the outer hips in.
- Reach the knees towards the right elbow. Move smoothly, and with control. As you take the legs over, lift the lower leg up slightly, so

that it supports the upper leg and controls the speed of the movement. Move the right ankle to the left ankle, the right knee to the left knee, the right thigh to the left thigh. At the same time, reach the left fingers away more.

- Turn your abdomen diagonally to the left hand.
- Draw the abdomen to the spine, bring the knees back to centre, then repeat to the other side.

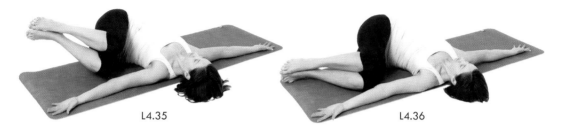

L4.35   L4.36

Jathara Parivartanasana, with legs straight

- Be in Pawanmuktasana, with the arms wide. Extend the fingers away. Straighten the legs so that the feet reach to the ceiling. Bring the feet towards the face a little, stretch the left hand away more, and bring the feet towards the right hand. Keep the lower leg resisting upward to control the speed at which you bring both legs down. Extend the top hip to the top foot, so that the feet stay together. When the feet touch the hand, engage the sacrum, draw the lower abdomen back to the spine and turn the abdomen away from the legs more. Turn the chest away from the legs.

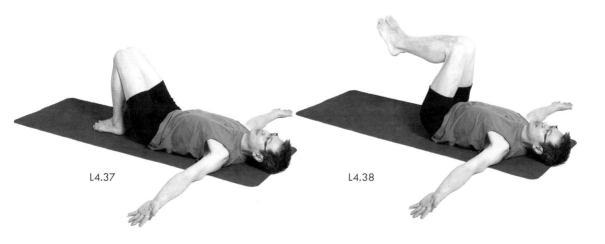

L4.37   L4.38

L4

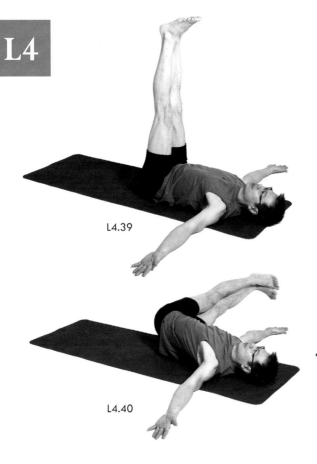

L4.39

L4.40

- Suck the abdomen in to bring the legs back to a vertical position, then go to the other side *(L4.41)*.
- Keep the face quiet and looking at the ceiling, and the shoulders away from the ears throughout.
- To finish, rest with the knees bent and the soles of the feet on the floor. Have the feet a little apart, so the knees fall against each other, allowing the abdomen to rest.
- If you choose, you can repeat this posture – on both the bent and straight leg versions – several times.

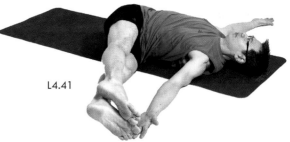

L4.41

Supta Swastikasana, with the feet supported

Supine cross-legged posture

- Lie down, as if for Savasana, but with the backs of the knees over a bolster or folded blanket. Release the shoulder muscles away from the ears so the chest is

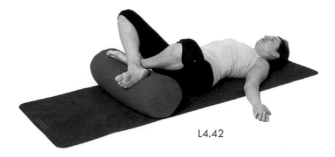

L4.42

L4

open, and move the flesh of the buttocks and the tailbone away from the waist so the spine is lengthened. From here, cross the legs so the feet rest on the support, and the knees release down. Rest the backs of the hands on the floor, or place the hands on the abdomen.

- After a few moments, release and change the cross of the legs.

Supta Baddha Konasana, with the feet supported

Supine bound angle pose

- Lie down as you did for Supta Swastikasana. Take the feet up on to the support, place the soles of the feet together, and extend the inner legs away so the outer knees release down. Lengthen the skin on the back of the head away from the shoulders, and soften the skin on the forehead down towards the eyebrows, and out to the temples.

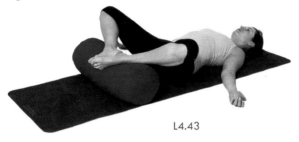

L4.43

Savasana

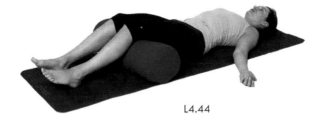

L4.44

A QUICK REMINDER

L4

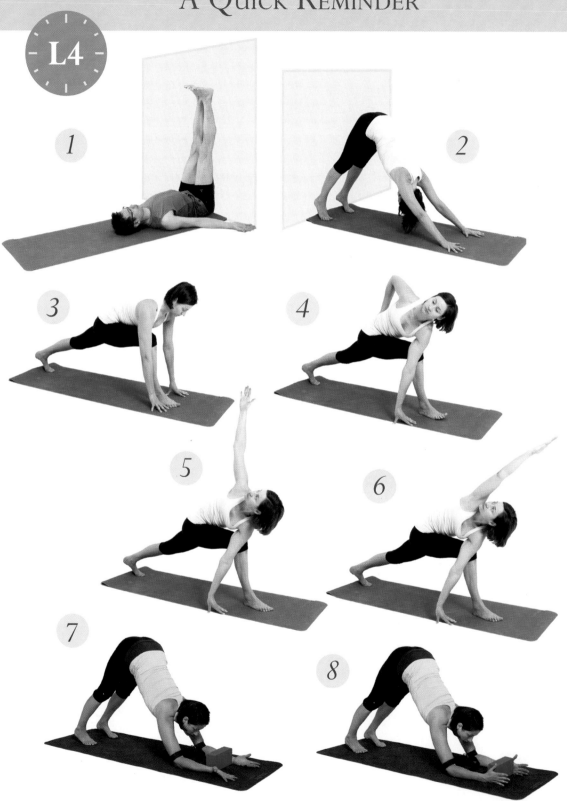

L4

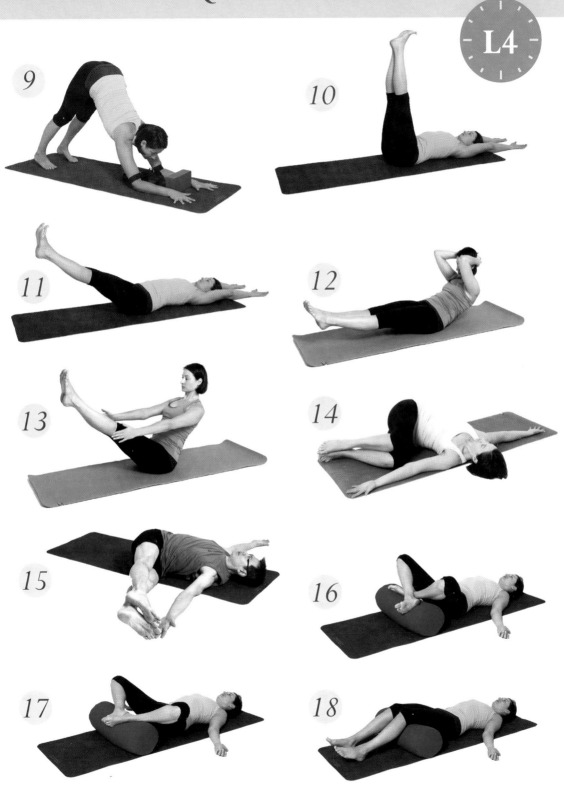

ACKNOWLEDGEMENTS

Thanks to Julie Hodges and Sheila Haswell, for their teaching, guidance and support.

Thanks to Ajay Parmar, for his constancy and clarity of thought and action.

Thanks to Rachel Wade.

Thanks to all my pupils.

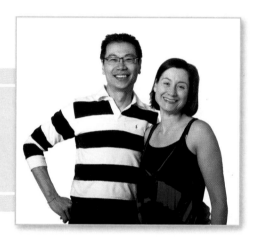

Thanks to **Peter Kosasih**, for his support, friendship and a shared yoga journey.

MANY THANKS

prAna clothing
for providing the men's yoga clothing shown throughout this book,
available at yogamatters – www.yogamatters.com

Sweaty Betty
for providing the women's yoga clothing shown throughout this book
www.sweatybetty.com

yogamatters
for providing the yoga equipment shown throughout this book
www.yogamatters.com